AN UNCOMMON DRUNK

AN UNCOMMON DRUNK

◆

Revelations of a High-Functioning Alcoholic

What You Don't Know Can Kill You

Jeff Herten, M.D.

iUniverse, Inc.

New York Lincoln Shanghai

AN UNCOMMON DRUNK
Revelations of a High-Functioning Alcoholic

Copyright © 2006 by R. Jeffrey Herten, M.D.

iUniverse books may be ordered through booksellers or by contacting:

iUniverse
2021 Pine Lake Road, Suite 100
Lincoln, NE 68512
www.iuniverse.com
1-800-Authors (1-800-288-4677)

ISBN-13: 978-0-595-37994-1 (pbk)
ISBN-13: 978-0-595-82365-9 (ebk)
ISBN-10: 0-595-37994-X (pbk)
ISBN-10: 0-595-82365-3 (ebk)

Printed in the United States of America

Contents

ACKNOWLEDGMENTS

I wrote this book to thank God for sparing the life of a dear friend: my horse, Famus. After making the commitment to write it, several people encouraged me, including my wife, Debby; friend, Charlene Price; colleague, Dr. Jim Reed; mentor Dr. Bud Beecher; and prayer partners John Maulhardt and Dan Weber. I am grateful to all of them for their support. A longtime friend, Jane Broshears, read my manuscript and volunteered to help get it published. Her skilled editing and deep belief in its message were instrumental in the completion of the final manuscript. I also would like to thank Kim Avalon for her secretarial help and Emily Higgins for her enthusiastic problem-solving skills.

I want to credit, most of all, my higher power, through whose strength I maintain sobriety and seek contentment. In the long process of writing and publishing this work, there were countless moments when things fell mysteriously into place, where the right idea or phrase or the right person materialized. Call them signs or omens, I choose to see them as evidence of a power greater than myself directing this work and ensuring its success.

For all of this, I am truly grateful.

rjh 10/3/05

INTRODUCTION

*"Supernatural joy is in no way that kind of dissipation, relaxation, and
license by which too many people try to forget their human dignity."*

—Mother Marie Des Douleurs

Ethyl alcohol, a simple hydrocarbon, is the most addictive drug on the
planet—not because it is the most pharmacologically addictive (though it may
be), but because it is the most accessible, macho, seductive, and legal drug available.

Why is it so addictive? Because, somewhere on the way to intoxication, there
is a brief moment when we feel *so good*. It is a feeling of well-being, of no worries
produced by the dissolution of inhibitions that alcohol effects. It is by removing
these inhibitions, these little anxieties that we tote, that alcohol works its magic.
It is the feeling we seek when we've had a grueling day at the office and want to
relax with a glass of wine. It is the emotionally "at ease" state we desire when we
enter a room full of intimidating people at a party and head directly for the bar. It
is the invigoration we strive for when we are emotionally exhausted and need a
boost. And it is the amusing, happy-go-lucky attitude that our friends enjoy in us
after we have had that first beer.

Unfortunately, that special feeling is fleeting. As we continue to drink, it disappears and is replaced by intoxication. Having experienced "the feeling," we
keep drinking, hoping that more alcohol will restore it. It doesn't. But we keep
trying. And in the process, we develop a psychological and physical dependence,
an addiction to this all-pervasive drug.

Alcohol is the most destructive drug on the planet. It has killed more people,
directly or indirectly, than anything else except war and plague. It is responsible
for more human misery than any other drug: more homicides, spousal and child
abuses, sexual assaults, traffic deaths, violent crimes, and diseases of abuse. Those
whose first addiction is alcohol often also become habituated to methamphetamine, cocaine, heroin, and prescription painkillers.

If alcohol were introduced today as a new product, its legal sales would be
fought vigorously. But it's not new. It's been around since Eve picked a slightly

fermented apple off the tree, fed it to Adam, and watched as he became giddy. Alcohol is so much a part of our society that it seems downright un-American to oppose it. What would a baseball game be without a beer? How can we eat a choice top sirloin without a good Cabernet?

So we succumb to our history, to peer pressure, and to effective media and marketing mind control. And we accept it. And we drink it. And slowly, insidiously, we become addicted. Alcohol morphs us into an unfamiliar character: a comedian who's the life of the party until he gets ridiculous and pathetic; a Romeo until he can't achieve an erection; a fearless superhero until he becomes aggressive and belligerent.

I grew up thinking that every family in America celebrated happy hour. Dad would come home after work and drink two stiff highballs. And on New Year's Day, friends would gather around the television for the Rose Parade and drink screwdrivers and Bloody Marys. For special occasions, there were gin fizzes and rum punches. Every occasion was built around or served as an excuse for consuming varying and increasing amounts of alcohol. It took me fifty-four years to come to my senses, to see alcohol as the mind-altering, addictive, health-destroying substance that it is. What a revelation!

So let me take you on my odyssey, which was the ever-narrowing maze of a deluded person who looked at life as a series of opportunities to celebrate anything and everything with a drink. Let me introduce you to some characters who shared my travels but who fell victim to the effects of the drug long before I did. I will describe what it's like to die of alcohol poisoning, in a one-night binge or from thirty years of hard drinking. You'll meet, among others, highly effective, successful, productive people who all have one terrible secret: they are drunk nearly every day, and they can't function without alcohol. These are the HFAs, the high-functioning alcoholics, and they comprise a large proportion of our society. Traditional wisdom alleges that 10 percent of men and 5 percent of women are hard-core alcoholics, the common drunks. Recent studies show that 30 percent of the U.S. population are "binge drinkers," in that they get drunk at least once a month. But there are no accurate statistics for high-functioning alcoholics because they are largely invisible in our culture, except to their spouses, children, and co-workers.

They are very uncommon drunks, but they are drunks just the same.

Allow me to present to you the scientific facts on the health hazards of alcohol, facts you've never heard or read before, facts the marketers of a multibillion-dollar industry don't want you to know. For example, regular alcohol intake increases the risk of developing cancer, osteoporosis, birth defects, allergies, and infections.

The alcohol industry has kept the truth from public awareness. Therefore, you may be shocked and amazed at your lack of information. But after reading this book, you will know the truth about alcohol.

I need to tell this story because, after more than thirty years, I am free. Free from the uncontrollable need to drink. Free from the despair of waking up every morning and knowing that I had again lost the battle against this addiction. Free from the certain disaster that was waiting for me and is waiting for every alcoholic, as the ever-tightening downward spiral sucks us into helpless, hopeless abandonment of dignity, reason, and sanity to a two-carbon poison called ethanol.

If this narrative awakens a single person heading for the abyss; prevents one needless traffic death, one episode of spousal or child abuse, or one case of cancer; or restores the dignity and humanity of a solitary soul, it will have served its purpose.

1

REALIZATION

As shadows lengthened across the valley, the early sunset brought bone-chilling cold to the desert. Even in winter, Death Valley is forbidding. It proved to be the perfect place for a reckoning.

I was tired. I had ridden fifty miles on my young horse, Tuggy, from Panamint Springs just west of Death Valley to the Saline Valley and back. It was New Year's Eve, and the party was in full swing. I had drunk five or six beers, and I was visiting with friends at a table in the big tent while the country and western band was on a break.

Some kids were seated with the backs of their chairs against the far end of our table. They were wrestling and giggling, and their chairs kept banging into the table, jarring it. Glasses bounced with the vibration, spilling wine and champagne. The kids looked over, recognized the nuisance they were creating, and kept right on wrestling.

Where were their parents? These kids didn't belong at an adult New Year's Eve party.

After another hard lurch of the table, I had had enough. I walked over to the kids and grabbed the nearest by the back of his neck, firmly. Startled, he squirmed away, rising from the chair. Tightening my grip, I forced him down into his chair and growled at him.

"You kids need to find another place to play."

As I loosened my grasp, he twisted away and was gone.

It was a dull party, and I left after a couple more beers. As I departed, fellow rider and longtime friend, Ellen, approached me.

"Do you know Tommy Holden?"

"Who is that?"

"A little boy. He says you grabbed him by the neck and hurt him. His neck is bruised."

"What?"

"He said some drunk grabbed him, and he pointed you out. I told his mom I would look into it." The words hit me like a slap in the face.

"Listen, Ellen, those kids were deliberately banging our table. I just sat him down. He squirmed away from me, so maybe the skin got pinched under his jacket."

"I saw his neck, Jeff. It's bruised."

"Ellen, I didn't mean to hurt the kid. I was only trying to get his attention."

"I'll talk to his mom and try to explain," Ellen offered.

I went to bed, but I didn't sleep. I couldn't believe that I hurt the boy; it seemed as if I'd barely touched him. I wasn't drunk. The seven or eight beers I drank were spread over five or six hours. Yet the fact remained, he was hurt. And I had done it.

I was sick with guilt and humiliation. What had he said? "Some drunk" grabbed him. I knew that there were times when alcohol made me angry, surly—but I had never hurt a child before. I saw myself through the eyes of that young boy: a big, mean drunk who grabbed him and slammed him into the chair. That was me.

In the morning, before the drive home, I had to meet with the boy's mother. All the denials in the world couldn't change the fact that his neck was bruised. I apologized feebly and prayed that the encounter would end. I didn't try to defend myself; my actions were indefensible. I listened to an outraged mother and just looked at the ground. Mercifully, it finally did end.

Alone on the long drive home, I experienced the most severe depression I have ever known. I was sick at heart, and I could understand why someone who felt this disconsolate could end their life. The psychological pain I experienced could become unbearable. In the silence of the truck, I carefully dissected all the circumstances that had brought me to the flash point. I was physically exhausted from riding 150 miles in the last four days. I had been taking ibuprofen for knee pain that resulted from the riding, and I had been, as usual, drinking. I had read that chronic ibuprofen use could cause severe depression, which certainly could have been a factor. The exhaustion contributed to it, I was sure. But, in the depths of my soul, I knew that the real cause was the alcohol and the losing battle that I had been waging to control it.

I had tried numerous times to quit. Every time I had failed. I felt so weak and flawed that I couldn't respect this person I had become. And now, I had let my addiction turn me into a physically assaultive person. I had hurt a child.

A common drunk. That's what I had become. I fantasized a video of me unsteady, slurring my words, bullying a child.

A common drunk. The realization of the truth was so revolting that I vowed this, finally, would be the experience that would make me quit.

And it did. I had a few beers once a week for the month of January, rationalizing as I had countless times before that I was in control, that I could drink once a week and leave it at that. But I knew deep inside that was a lie. I knew within a couple of months I would be drinking three days a week, then five. And within six months, I would resume the pattern of near daily consumption. I knew, for me, it was all or nothing.

It had to be nothing.

Lent approached. The practice of giving up something for Lent has, at times, been trivialized. In the early Christian Church, Lent was a time of somber introspection and rigorous fasting, a ritual sharing of Jesus's suffering. The sacrifice should be of consequence: something precious and desirable that distracts us from our spiritual focus. Alcohol certainly was that for me. I prayed for the strength to quit, knowing that with my will alone, it could not be done.

My prayer was answered. A strength beyond my own was there, and still is.

Four months later, I experienced a miracle that could never have occurred when I was drinking. It made it possible for some remarkable veterinarians to save the life of a horse I dearly love, my magnificent bay gelding, Famus.

My wife, Debby, and I were part of a group riding the historic Pony Express Trail from Missouri to California. A month into the ride, on a blistering hot day in Wyoming, Famus's intestines shut down. The resultant colic caused him unbearable pain and he stretched as if to pee and pawed the ground frantically trying to ease his suffering.

The vets attending the ride treated him for over six hours with no improvement. They made it very clear that if I couldn't get him more aggressive care, the poisons fermenting in his stagnant gut would destroy his kidneys within hours.

The only option was a four-hour trailer ride to the Veterinary School at Colorado State. It was an hour before midnight.

In my drinking days I would have had four or five beers by then and been unfit to drive. Even though exhausted from an eight-hour ride in the heat, I was sober and committed to saving this very special friend.

I did, or rather, the vets did. Two days later, I returned to the ride, leaving behind a convalescing but healthy Famus. I didn't leave behind the memory of a long night of prayer to the same power that gave me the strength to quit drinking, and the calm certainty that came over me, reassuring me that he would live.

On the long drive northward, I thanked God that he had given me the presence of mind and the sobriety to save him. As my eyes filled with tears of gratitude, I got a clear message that I could express my thanks in tangible form if I would share my story with others. In a nearly four-decade-long struggle, I had finally learned the truth about alcohol. I am free, no longer a slave to alcohol. It neither owns nor controls me anymore. My newfound freedom has provided me undeniable peace and contentment. I look back on those dark days of addiction and marvel at what a blessing it is to be sober. Yet I see so many people who are struggling as I was, and I want to help them experience the joy of real freedom from addiction. It was time for me to share my story with others deluded as I was, suffering as I was, denying as I was.

I made a promise that day on the drive north to Casper. It has taken me over four years, but I have kept it. Every time I got tired or discouraged, I'd look out in the pasture and see that gorgeous bay gelding, remember that miracle, and get writing again.

Since I quit, I have gained some remarkable insights into the insidious and pervasive disease that alcohol has become for so many individuals, and for our society as a whole. It has truly been an awakening.

This book will relate my story and the story of others who became addicted to alcohol. In every case, alcohol fulfilled a need. Perhaps, in reading these stories, you may see a similarity to the way you use alcohol. Possibly, you will come to understand that alcohol is often used as a coping mechanism. Unfortunately, it doesn't work very well and produces a multitude of negative side effects, the worst and most common, that it is highly addictive. So, even if you do finally realize that it is not helping you cope, it's often too late. You're already hooked. An additional negative consequence of looking for an external fix is that you never dig deep enough and find the source of power within that can handle anything. Discovering that strength can be a life-altering experience rewarded by peace and self-satisfaction.

Does sobriety seem like an unattainable goal? It's not. The wonderful news is that it is never too late to change. Freedom from alcoholism is possible. It requires knowledge, understanding, and resolve. This book is designed to provide the first two and to help you or your loved one find the last.

Let's get started.

This is my prayer: that my success in overcoming my alcohol addiction might help you to acknowledge and overcome yours, or that it might help a loved one who needs to know the truth about their problem and resolve to change.

2

YOU'RE DIFFERENT WHEN YOU DRINK

○ ○

"There was once a gypsy saying,
It came from Catalan:
First the man he takes the drink
And then the drink it takes the man."

—*Tom Russell*

You might have inferred from the last chapter that I was a serious alcoholic. I wasn't. I never got sloppy drunk. I never got sick, never fell down, and rarely felt bad the next day. I never drank during the day. I would never dream of drinking at lunch and going back to work. I never drank myself senseless or went on a binge. I was a well-respected physician in my community and taught on the faculty of the medical school. I never clouded my judgment with alcohol.

Until the workday was over.

Then I would stop off at the local liquor store and pick up a six-pack of one of my favorite beers. I would crack one just after I turned up the country lane on which I live, and I had it down before I reached my driveway just over two miles up the road. I enjoyed the cold, refreshing taste, but the speed with which I drank it reveals that I was doing it for one reason: how it made me feel.

I would drink a second beer as I fed the horses, and that warm euphoria would ooze through me. Inwardly, there would be a long sigh as all the cares of the day faded away. But the feeling would be fleeting, and I tried to regain it with another beer at dinner and sometimes another after that. If you phoned after dinner, you might hear a little slurring at the edge of my speech. I became self-conscious about it and would rarely call anyone or answer the phone after dinner.

I functioned at a very high level most of the time. I didn't consume that much, but I drank almost every day. I was addicted to alcohol, and it ruled my life. I refer to myself as a high-functioning alcoholic. There are millions of us. You may be one.

So what's the harm? People like me are not a menace to society. We just have a few drinks after work to unwind. No harm there.

At first, maybe. My dad was like that. Every night he came home and had two double scotches or bourbons or vodka and tonics; the liquor depended on whatever phase he and Mom were in. It seemed innocent enough. But at the dinner table more and more often he would become argumentative. He would single someone out, usually my sister, Julie, and pick a fight with her. It didn't matter about what. And he would pursue it until he had insulted and ridiculed her in front of the rest of the family.

Sober, my dad wasn't like that. He was one of the sweetest, most loving and sentimental people on earth. So, how could he so readily demean his daughter? He couldn't. It wasn't him. It was the alcohol.

This scene is repeated thirty million times at dinner tables all over America. Kids stare at their dinner plates, afraid to look up and become the target. In many households, it's not an argument: it's a brawl. Some poor kid gets slapped, punched, or slammed against a wall. God forbid, the baby is a little colicky and begins to cry. A drinking dad may not have the patience for that. Statistics show alcohol is involved in over 50 percent of child abuse incidents. Often, these are otherwise good dads who hold down jobs and support and love their families. But alcohol changes them, makes them angry, shortens their fuse, and diminishes their impulse control. And so they shake that crying baby or slap that whining child. It is not really who they are; it is who they are with two gin and tonics or four beers in them. But the injured and frightened child doesn't know that. All he knows is that his home is a place of senseless fear and pain.

Many angry and abusive dads and moms are not your textbook alcoholics. A large proportion of them are like me. They function well in society, have successful careers, and are well-respected members of the community. But they still drink too much too often, causing problems for their families and themselves. They are high-functioning alcoholics, like me. But they are alcoholics just the same.

Is there such a thing as harmless drinking? Am I completely opposed to alcohol? I know that I am totally opposed to alcohol for me and for others like me. I have an addictive personality. It took me fifty-four years to come to the awareness that I cannot drink, even a little bit, without it becoming a problem. And for a significant proportion of drinkers, I think that is true. Are there people who can just have a glass of wine at night and not have it get them eventually into trouble? There are, but I believe they are far fewer than we expect. If they drink wine, what are they drinking for? For the nose? The wonderful aroma of fermented grapes that can take on such amazing subtlety and complexity? Perhaps, but in order to taste and compare a number of wines, one has to consume a significant amount of alcohol. Certainly, some can handle it without being drawn into the downward spiral that is addiction, but a substantial percentage cannot; it just fuels the growing problem.

It is a very individual situation, and only that particular person knows, if he is truly honest with himself, whether he drinks for taste and aroma or if he drinks for the effect the alcohol has on his brain. If it is the latter, then he has the potential to get into trouble. Statistics vary and it is impossible to arrive at an accurate number, but as much as a third of all people who consume alcohol will develop a problem with it (Jefferis 2005).

I was a part of that third.

Are you?

3

HOW ALCOHOL MAKES YOU DRUNK

Pop the cap off that Budweiser and take a long slow drink. Ice-cold and refreshing, the beer flows into your mouth and down your throat along with alcohol, the two-carbon chemical sought in an almost infinite variety by nearly every culture on the globe. Before it even reaches your stomach, it enters your bloodstream as you can feel the very first signs of a warm mellowness that you have grown to love. Alcohol is unusual in that it is absorbed right through the mucosa, the lining of your mouth, esophagus, and stomach. It is such a small molecule that it doesn't have to be broken down by any digestive enzymes and thus passes directly through the wall of any portion of the gut. This is in distinct contrast to most foods containing the three major energy sources: carbohydrates, proteins, and fats. Most of these are large complex molecules that must be broken down into smaller molecular fragments by stomach acid or by digestive enzymes in the mouth or small intestine to be absorbed. Absorption of alcohol begins immediately after that first swallow and continues until the last two-carbon fragment is absorbed in the small intestine. Unlike many foods and most medications, alcohol is 100 percent absorbed into the bloodstream, and quickly and evenly distributed to all organs of the body, muscles, fat, and, of course, the brain.

Since alcohol is so chemically simple, the body assimilates it very quickly. Its small size and simple structure allows it to pass readily through the membrane of every cell in the body. Alcohol functions as a two-carbon sugar, so it is considered to be in the carbohydrate family. It is metabolized preferentially over glucose in the liver and converted to a chemical called acetaldehyde at a fixed rate of one ounce per hour. Acetaldehyde is a toxic, cancer-causing chemical, and it is the toxicity that is responsible for a large portion of the damage alcohol does to the body. The higher the blood alcohol is, the higher the acetaldehyde concentration.

Alcohol is a cell poison. At high concentrations it interferes with normal cell metabolism and is toxic to many cells in the body, including the liver, heart, and nervous system.

Although the temporary effect of alcohol may be pleasurable, it has many damaging effects on your body. The ounce and a half of alcohol in that Budweiser will be well-traveled before it is passed into your urine or breathed out in an exhalation. It is illuminating to see where it has been in the interim.

A small amount is absorbed through the linings (mucosae) of the mouth, esophagus, and stomach. The majority is absorbed in the upper part of the small intestine. This portion of the small bowel is responsible for the absorption of many of the vitamins that are necessary for normal bodily function. Alcohol partially inhibits that absorption, causing alcoholics to be deficient in crucial vitamins. These vitamin deficiencies produce many of the long-term deleterious effects of alcoholism. The principal cause of vitamin deficiencies in alcoholics is that, being drunk much of the time, they ignore their diets. Many do not have the intake of vital nutrients essential for normal cell functions, especially the cells of the central nervous system.

Once absorbed, the alcohol is carried into small veins in the wall of the intestine, which coalesce into larger veins, eventually forming the large portal vein that carries the ethanol and all other digested and absorbed nutrients to the liver to be processed. Everything that is ingested orally must first pass through the liver before being distributed to the rest of the body. Thus, the liver is the most vulnerable to the toxic effect of alcohol and all other poisons. The liver alters what it can of the alcohol, breaking it down to acetaldehyde, but it can handle only an ounce an hour, so the overflow enters the general circulation to intoxicate the rest of the tissues. Alcohol is an equal opportunity intoxicant. It poisons all cells to the same degree. It's just that some cells, like nerve tissue, are much more sensitive and prone to damage than others. Fat is relatively insensitive because alcohol is not very soluble in it. Fat does have a large reservoir of blood vessels, however, and the effect of dilution of a larger blood volume allows higher doses of alcohol with relatively lower blood alcohol level. Nevertheless, all tissues are affected. Alcohol is soluble in the aqueous world of our tissues, so it passes readily into every cell.

Alcohol has the most notable effect on the nervous system. This system functions by an interchange, release, and reuptake of a number of chemical messages that are highly complex and not fully understood. When alcohol enters a nerve cell, it alters the amount of the chemical message the nerve cell releases, and it also changes the reuptake of those chemicals that are critical for their normal functioning. Very quickly there develops a dependence on the presence of alcohol in order for the chemical message to be released.

In low concentrations, alcohol is a mild stimulant, and it may have a slight antianxiety effect as well, allowing individuals to feel invigorated and notice freedom from social inhibitions. Alcohol is a great "social lubricant," as it fosters in shy people with mild social anxiety the ability to feel more relaxed in what would otherwise be anxiety-provoking situations.

The alcohol circulating in the blood is carried to the kidneys. Here, it inhibits a naturally occurring substance called antidiuretic hormone (ADH), producing a brisk diuresis or increase in urine production. Beer drinkers have to urinate a lot not just because of the volume of beer that they drink but also because alcohol is a diuretic. Chronic alcoholism can cause dehydration of all the cells in the body, a fact that makes drinking and exercising in hot weather dangerous for the unwary. Hot tubs can also be hazardous for both the acute and chronically intoxicated person. Already dehydrated with a low blood volume, the alcoholic dehydrates further in the heat of the tub. If the blood volume gets critically low, blood pressure may plummet, causing the parboiled drunk to pass out and possibly drown. There are more than a few accidental deaths due to intoxicated hot-tubbers.

Alcohol may also cause the kidney to excrete more calcium due to increased urine production. The speeded-up flow of urine prevents the kidney tubules from reabsorbing calcium. Alcohol also increases urinary loss of calcium by altering levels of parathyroid hormone that are responsible for its conservation. Chronic alcohol intake leads to a long-term loss of bone density.

Acute intoxication causes muscle cell death as a result of the toxic effect of ethanol on muscle. Alcoholic myonecrosis may be mild, but in severe cases, enough myoglobin, the large oxygen-carrying protein in muscle cells analogous to hemoglobin, may be released from dying muscle cells to stain the urine a vin-rose color. The myoglobin can even plug millions of tiny little filter apparatuses or glomeruli in the kidneys and produce kidney failure. Chronic alcoholism leads to muscle shrinkage or atrophy and to weakness.

Since the heart is a muscle, it is vulnerable to the toxic effects of alcohol as well. Long-term exposure produces an alcoholic cardiomyopathy, which weakens the heart and can produce congestive heart failure.

As it circulates through the body, alcohol produces a mild dilation of blood vessels, especially in the skin. This produces the flushed face of the acutely intoxicated and may contribute to the large dilated veins seen on the cheeks and nose of many drinkers. To be fair, there are many other factors contributing to the facial veins such as heredity, sun, and diet, but there is little question that if a person is predisposed to this problem, alcohol use will aggravate it.

The dilation of skin blood vessels caused by alcohol may result in a prompt and dramatic heat loss as the warm blood, reaching the surface, radiates heat into the surrounding environment. People who are acutely intoxicated are at great risk of hypothermia in a cold environment because they are losing heat to the air and alcohol decreases their sensitivity to the effects of the cold. This accounts for the death of many alcoholics from "exposure" each winter.

When considering the many short- and long-term effects of alcohol, two questions arise. First, why isn't educating the public a higher priority for health-care professionals? Second, once people are educated, will they continue to drink and if they do, why? Hopefully, the information in this book will help to answer these and other questions. Perhaps it will convince you to rethink your present drinking habits and/or those of your friends and loved ones.

4

MY LIFE WITH THE BOTTLE PART I

Beer is one of my oldest friends. My first recollection of drinking was sitting on the front lawn with my dad after he'd finished mowing the lawn and getting a sip of the beer he quaffed on a hot summer afternoon. It was Olympia, and the fizzy bubbles tickled my nose. The taste was bitter but with a subtle hidden tingle. I learned to love that taste. When I started drinking beer in earnest in college and later, it never tasted the same, or as good, as it did on those hot summer Saturdays. I was eight years old. I never got more than a single sip, so I am sure I was never intoxicated, but special times with Dad became associated with drinking.

They were called "French 75's," named for the storied cannons of World War I. Made from champagne and brandy, poured in a tulip-stem glass, they were my first real taste of alcohol. I was about fifteen. We were at our neighbor's, the McDougalls, for a Christmas open house. Jack McDougall decided that the kids would be allowed to try one. We were each given our own glass of the sparkling elixir. I remember feeling the bubbles all the way down my throat and up my nose, but I liked the taste. A half hour later I had the most peculiar sensation. I felt warm all over. A gentle heat started at the top of my head and spread slowly down across my face, neck, torso, and out to the tips of my fingers. It proceeded all the way to the bottoms of my feet, which itched in an odd way. It felt very strange but good, like the world was smiling; everything was okay. A little while later I felt fuzzy. My vision was slightly blurred. I was momentarily frightened, but then it passed. I was experiencing the effect of alcohol for the first time.

There was a myth when I was in high school that two aspirin and a Coke would make you tipsy. I tried it on a youth group weekend retreat at Yosemite trying to impress a young lady with how sophisticated and cool I was. Although it didn't work, I acted intoxicated anyway. She was not impressed. It's interesting now to reflect on how important and mature I was trying to feel by getting intoxicated. Sadly, I had already learned some lessons from my family life about the importance of altering my mood with alcohol to feel good.

My best friend in high school was a bright, sarcastic, and worldly boy named George Townes. We had been on a debate team together in Forensic League and were also members of the same high school YMCA club. George had a wonderful sense of humor and was fun to be around. He also had a drinking problem. George's parents were both in the motion picture business and, like my parents, they drank heavily and saw no problem with George drinking along with them. They were gone often, especially on weekends, and George would help himself to their bourbon or scotch and take me for a ride in his Plymouth with the push-button transmission. There were some hair-raising rides on the narrow, winding roads of the Hollywood hills, lurching around tight corners and screaming along straight stretches of Mulholland Drive at ninety miles an hour. It's a wonder we weren't killed, but the thought never entered my mind. I was just exhilarated. I did not drink then. I was a late bloomer socially and rather straight, but I did enjoy my crazy friend.

George went off to the University of Washington and continued his drinking unabated. In his freshman year, at a fraternity party, he drank himself almost unconscious and, stumbling out of the party, he slipped on some ice and struck his head on solid concrete. He was in a coma for just shy of a week, and when he recovered, he couldn't remember his class schedule or how to drive to the campus. Eventually, it all came back, but it scared him into never drinking again. George is now a professor of English at a major university. Sober.

Similarly, college almost killed me. Literally. I was seventeen years old, socially very immature and suddenly alone in a culture where alcohol was venerated, almost worshipped. It began the summer before my freshman year with fraternity rush parties: poolside gatherings at fabulous homes in Palos Verdes or dances in funky beer halls near campus. The prospective pledges were sure to be introduced to the big-name athletes of each house. And there was lots of beer. I was cautious about drinking more than a couple of glasses. I had never really been drunk, and I didn't want to create a negative impression, as drinking was still a mysterious and unexplored journey for me. I had watched my parents for years, so I knew how people acted when they drank. I had also observed my uncle who was always sloppy drunk and rude at holiday family gatherings, but I hadn't had the experience firsthand, so I was very tentative. The fraternities were careful not to let the rush party drinking get too out of hand. The hardcore drinkers were warned about getting drunk and insulting the rushees. Instead, they paraded all their athletes, student leaders, and notable alumni by us during these parties: handsome clean-cut guys in button-down shirts. But there was always the beer. And there was no question that we were expected to drink it. No one abstained at these functions. I don't remember a single person at any of these parties, male or female, that didn't drink.

I immediately joined a fraternity that was well stocked with all-American swimmers, golfers, and trackmen; a house that was considered very cool by my sister, a member of one of the better sororities on campus. Sadly, I didn't pick the group of young men by any criteria other than the reputation they had around campus, and I didn't wait several semesters to really assess what was happening in the Greek system. I was young and insecure, and I wanted a social anchor in the very imposing university life I was beginning. So I pledged.

Several weeks after the end of rush, the house had a big party. A bus was hired to take a large group out to a small lake on the outskirts of the city. Several of the upperclassmen had driven down to Mexico to buy gallons of "white lightning," 99 percent ethanol. Placed in grape and lime Kool-Aid and poured into empty beer kegs, it became "Purple Passion" and "Green Death." Members, pledges, and their dates filed onto the bus and the party and the drinking began immediately. I drove separately because my date was an old high school girlfriend who was just beginning her senior year and I had to pick her up at home.

We had a little trouble finding the venue, and by the time we arrived, the party was in full swing. A band played on a large swath of grass along the shore. There were a few couples dancing while many sat around the lawn and listened. And drank. I knew what was in the punch and warned my date not to drink too much. Many were uninformed or unwise. Several hours, a sunken canoe, a broken rope swing, and untold numbers of retches later, forty couples staggered back to the bus and headed for campus. When they arrived back at the fraternity, the sides of the bus were decorated with vomit: chunks of pineapple with faint green and purple streaks.

I drank several of the punches but didn't feel drunk. My date, a little tipsy, snoozed on my arm as I drove home. Just as I reached the freeway, brilliant red lights appeared in my rearview mirror. A cold fear gripped me as a spotlight illuminated the interior of the car. I rolled down the window and a highway patrolman shined a light in my face.

"May I see your driver's license?"

"Yes sir. Is there a problem officer?" I handed him my opened wallet.

"Please take it out." I removed it and handed it to him.

"Did you know you had a taillight out?"

"No sir. It's my dad's car and I only drive it on weekends."

He handed the license back to me.

"Were you at the party at the lake?"

"Yes sir."

"Have you been drinking?"

"Yes sir."

He studied me for a long minute. I was seventeen years old. Any drinking at my age was illegal, let alone driving under the influence.

"You better be going straight home, young man."

"Yes sir." He turned and strode back to his patrol car as I wilted in a sigh of relief.

This was 1965. The no-tolerance policy for alcohol that exists now was years in the future. A kindly man took pity on a basically good kid and let him go. I wonder how different my life would have been had I been cited. A 502 on my record might have ruined my chances for medical school. I was definitely the recipient of a gift of grace that night. Too bad I was too young to experience the awakening that I did when Tommy Holden labeled me "some drunk" at that New Year's Eve party. But I couldn't imagine all the misery that alcohol would bring to friends and acquaintances, and to me. I had no insight, no point of reference other than my upbringing in a drinking family. No one prompted me to question whether this was sane or healthy behavior. So rather than learn a lesson, I felt I'd had a very close call. I learned not to drive with burned-out taillights, to use backstreets and out-of-the-way routes to get home when I had been drinking. Through the grace of God, I never have been stopped or cited for driving under the influence.

The next day, I bragged to my fraternity brothers about being stopped. I was typical of many young people, both then and now. Young adults are at risk for two major reasons. First, they so desperately want to be accepted by their peer group that they will do almost anything. Witness the popularity of tattoos and piercings, or the violent and inhumane acts that adolescent gang members will perform to be part of the group. Drinking and drinking to excess is another ritual that young (and not so young) people partake of to be accepted. Second, young adults have no sense of their mortality. They feel totally invincible; thus they partake in many high-risk behaviors such as drinking, driving fast, having unprotected sex, using illicit drugs, smoking cigarettes, and doing stunts such as diving off bridges into shallow rivers. Boys, of course, are the worst. Part of it is the testosterone, which fuels aggressive behavior, coupled with a lack of maturity in adolescent boys. A fascinating recent study showed that the male brain does not fully mature until the early-to-mid-twenties, providing some explanation for the dangerous and irrational behavior of teenage boys (CDC Fact Book 2001–2002).

My college fraternity fostered institutionalized alcoholism. The Christmas party was a perfect example. After picking the name of a brother out of a hat, each fraternity member bought that person a gift—invariably booze. One of the upperclassmen, dressed up as Santa Claus, arrived at the party already inebriated. Very few Santas made it through the Christmas party without passing out or throwing up, or both. At the party, Santa would pick a gift, read the tag, call the recipient up, and have him sit on Santa's knee while opening it. Then, the recipient had to drink it. Most of the time, the gift was hard liquor. Tequila was particularly popular. Mescal was too, especially Cusano Rojo, a large square yellow liquid-filled bottle with a hideous coiled red worm at the bottom. The challenge was to take a big chug and to swallow the worm.

My drinking skills made me somewhat of a legend one Christmas when I chugged a gallon of red wine. The cheap and popular Red Mountain came in gallon jugs. I chugged half of it, went outside and stuck my finger down my throat, vomited the first half, and then came back to finish it off. I vomited most of the second half also, but not enough to avoid a horrific headache the next day during my Inorganic Chemistry quiz.

Given the large amount of hard stuff that was consumed, it was a wonder that no one died of acute alcohol poisoning. It is very simple to kill yourself by drinking. If you consume alcohol faster than your body can metabolize it and you don't get sick and vomit before it reaches a toxic level in your blood stream and brain, you can die. It happens several dozen times a year on college campuses.

Amazingly, my college drinking experiences were considered entirely socially acceptable. It was the norm. Everybody drank themselves into a stupor on Friday and Saturday night. There may have been fraternity brothers who didn't drink as much, but they didn't let on because their peers might view them as "wimps." It was accepted that brothers and occasionally their dates would pass out at a party. I remember a party in the foothills one night when I took a drunken brother home in the trunk of my parents' car. Upon arrival at the fraternity house, he was still unconscious and had vomited all over the floor of the trunk. He could have easily aspirated the vomit and choked to death. But he didn't and everybody thought it was cool. Again, we were saved by a guardian angel who must have been shaking his head and praying we would learn from the experience and not put ourselves in harm's way again. We did not.

Sometime late in my sophomore year, my girlfriend and I broke up. In a ritual observance of grief, I publicly drank myself unconscious. It was a night of open houses on fraternity and sorority row, and I carried a half-gallon of "Spanada" (a poor attempt to re-create sangria) with me as I accompanied friends to the other houses. I remember tripping over a privet hedge and falling down at some point in the evening and barely making it back to my fraternity house before I passed out.

I awoke the next morning, lying fully clothed on my bed, covered with vomitus in varying stages of drying. I remembered nothing of getting sick. I didn't know then that a common secondary cause of death in acute alcohol poisoning is aspiration pneumonia, a process where corrosive stomach acid and enzymes are inhaled or aspirated into the lungs of stuporous or comatose individuals. These potent chemicals literally digest lung tissue, producing large pockets of necrotic tissue and pus. There is no satisfactory treatment for aspiration pneumonia, and if it isn't fatal, it often destroys large amounts of healthy lung tissue and leaves its victims respiratory cripples with diminished lung volumes and recurrent infections. Again, my guardian angel somehow turned my head to the side so the vomit decorated my pillow instead of filling my bronchi. I had no idea how lucky I had been until years later. I studied aspiration pneumonia in medical school and, when I was an intern, treated two cases. They were fatal. I had a long-term reminder of the incident, however. Some of the vomit had splattered on my shoes, a pair of oxblood Florsheim Imperial wingtips that my dad bought me when I left for college. The acid vomitus had digested away the shiny veneer and left dull spots that would never take a shine again. I had those shoes for twenty years, the dull spots reminding me of my alcoholic brush with death.

It was both a blessing and a curse that I tolerated alcohol well. I am a moderately tall guy and I was a little chunky, which was helpful since alcohol is evenly distributed in all tissues. Even though it is not very soluble in fat, adipose tissue is richly supplied with blood vessels, effectively diluting the alcohol, lowering the blood alcohol level and thus the effective dose. Big people, fat or not, can drink a great deal more, with less effect, than their small, thin counterparts. But, in my case, there was more to it than that. I could match a friend who was the same size and body fat beer for beer and not act as drunk. I was just as drunk as he, but something about my nervous system allowed me to function better with the same blood alcohol. I could hold my liquor and I was proud of that fact.

I functioned well after considerable alcohol intake, driving in a perfectly acceptable manner. When I had a great deal to drink, I would see double. That could make driving difficult. No problem. I found that by closing one eye, I had monocular vision again and drove merrily and relatively straight down the road. This was the 1960s and the police and highway patrol were not as vigilant as they are today. The real menace of drunk drivers was not as well understood or publicized in those days. I, and many of my college peers, got away with it.

Another of my college drinking exploits occurred in a high-class bar and restaurant a few blocks from campus frequented by alumni, staff, and occasionally undergraduates. Behind the bar, neatly arranged in wooden holders, were long glass beakers that measured eighteen or thirty-six inches: the fabled half-yard and yard of ale popularized by our cultural, political, and alcoholic ancestors, the Brits. There were periodic contests to see who could chug a yard (2.3 quarts) of ale the fastest, and anyone, at any time, could challenge the record. A decent time for a yard was five seconds, while most average beer drinkers might put it down in nine or ten seconds and be pleased. I had the questionable fortune of having the ability to open my throat and literally pour the beer down, while also possessing a rather large stomach volume. When I graduated from college, I held the record of 2.9 seconds for a yard: a dubious honor. Thirty-five years later, I wish my academic accomplishments had been as outstanding.

Additionally, in the 1960s, the concept of the addictive personality was known to the medical and psychiatric community, but it wasn't well-known to the general public. If it were, perhaps I would have recognized the signs in myself. Besides, I was no different from 80 percent of the guys in my fraternity. These were my peers, and they all drank hard. I desperately wanted to be one of them. I didn't know anyone who abstained from alcohol. If I had, I would have thought they were nerds. I drank no more than the majority of my fraternity brothers and a lot less than some. What I didn't realize was that we were all alcoholics in training. Sadly, most of us succeeded as high-functioning alcoholics and, a tragic few, as terminal drunks.

In my junior year, I was asked by a fellow student to tutor him in philosophy. I was a decent student, getting by more on intelligence than study habits, having been seduced by all the distractions of college life. He was the son of a famous actor, was wealthier than most of our peers, and was a very big man on campus. I was flattered to be asked.

We agreed to meet the night before the exam and "cram." He picked me up and we drove to his parents' opulent home in Brentwood. We began to study. By eleven o'clock it was obvious we could never cover the material in time for the exam. That's when Doug pulled out several small yellow pills, handed me one, and said, "This will help keep us alert to finish the job." I didn't ask what it was but I'm sure it was amphetamine, a potent stimulant and performance enhancer.

We studied all through the night. The mental focus produced by the drug was quite remarkable. Philosophy had never been this interesting before.

When I wrote the exam the next day, I filled two blue books and could have filled more. I earned the highest grade in the class. Doug got a B and was very pleased. I was amazed at the effect of this little yellow pill on my intellectual performance. It was a pharmacological epiphany.

Several postgraduate dental students still frequented the fraternity, occasionally for meals or a social event. In a casual conversation over a bridge game one evening, one of them intimated that most of the dental students took uppers to study. Could he get me some? Yes, indeed. My addiction to amphetamines began as simply as that.

I was involved in a great many student activities in college. Then a poor manager of time and a natural procrastinator, it was easy to put my studies on the back burner. I did go to class most of the time, but I did only a portion of the considerable reading that my classes required. It was easy to put off studying until the night before the exam, knowing I had a wonder pill that would allow me to cram three months of studying into an "all-nighter" and to perform extremely well on the exam.

The last year and a half of college, I used "speed" to study. The drug of choice was called Eskatrol. It was a prescription diet pill containing dexamphetamine sulfate combined with a very mild tranquilizer to mitigate the shakiness and anxiety side effect of the upper. It was amazing stuff, producing six to eight hours of intense concentration and total recall. By graduation from college, I couldn't study without it.

On a warm spring afternoon at the end of my senior year, I used up two more of my nine lives. I was in emotional turmoil: elated since I had just received my acceptance to medical school and greatly disturbed because the house-mother of the sorority where I worked serving meals, a dear friend, had suffered a massive stroke. I was hosting a mixer between the senior men's honor-service organization and a similar women's organization from the nearby Catholic university at my off-campus apartment. The party was in full swing and the beer was flowing freely. The club members were all well-oiled and pretty rowdy when Rudy, the apartment manager, arrived to investigate the commotion. I saw him coming down the drive and worked my way across the patio to intercept him but I was too late. Unaware who he was, one of the members had thrown a cup of beer at the intruder.

Rudy stomped down the drive. I probably should have pursued him and tried to assuage his anger, but I was drunk and having fun, and I figured he would get over it. I could apologize for my friends tomorrow.

I was at the hors d'oeuvres table when I sensed everyone turning toward the drive. There was Rudy, at the edge of the patio, holding a small pistol in the face of his tormenter. I was just drunk enough to have no fear. Rudy would never shoot anyone. He's just salving his pride, frightening this rude drunk. I moved unsteadily across the patio and stepped between them.

Now the gun was in my face, but I was too drunk to be frightened. I apologized for my intoxicated friend and hardly took note of the blue steel barrel waving in front of my nose. Rudy made a good show of it, insisting that I get out of the way so he could teach that "cabron" a lesson. Maybe he wouldn't shoot, but he was angry, the gun was loaded, and anything can happen when alcohol and firearms are involved. It was well-known around the complex that Rudy had a drinking problem, so how did I know he wasn't drunk enough to do something stupid? I didn't, but luckily, even drunk, I made the right call. After listening to my apologies for what seemed like an eternity but was probably only a minute or two, he put the gun back in his coat pocket and walked down the drive.

When the mixer was over, I performed a cursory cleanup and decided to head downtown to the Pantry for dinner. I enlisted a friend and we hopped into my '57 Volkswagen bug. Miraculously, we both put on our seat belts.

I had not consumed any beer for an hour or more, but I was still feeling the half dozen glasses I'd had at the party. I drove onto the freeway and got up to speed, moving over to the left for the transition road that would head north into the city. I was chatting with my friend when a car full of very attractive young ladies passed us on the right. Stan and I were very interested and attentive and the girls were clearly enjoying the high-speed encounter. I beeped my squeaky little horn, and as I did, I looked up to see the concrete railing of the tight turn of the transition road. With the distraction, I had not been paying attention and had failed to brake at the approach of the turn. I looked down to see seventy miles per hour registering on the speedometer, and as I looked up, the only object in my vision was a large yellow sign with the word "SLOW" and an arrow curving to the left.

Even the quick reflexes of a twenty-year-old could not slow the Beetle quickly enough to handle the tight curve. I braked hard and steered left but the bug skidded to the right. Sliding across the lane, I saw the concrete rail looming ahead. I corrected back to the right and the bug responded by skidding to the left. The railing on the other side loomed up. I steered back to the right. The rear end of the VW whipped around and now I found myself in a four-wheel drift back the other way. I tried to correct yet again but the torque was too much and the bug flipped. Everything seemed to be in slow motion inside the vehicle. I felt my door popping open and books and odd papers rained down and flew back again as we continued to roll. I counted two revolutions and then a slam as the chassis came to rest against the right side railing. Stan and I were hanging upside down, held in by the seat belts. Both doors had popped open and, without restraints, we would have certainly been ejected and crushed by the rolling vehicle.

The adrenaline produced by the crash and the fear of being caught created an urgency and a sobriety that saved us. Stan and I unfastened our belts, fell to the ceiling-now-floor, and climbed out. The front bonnet had popped open and the spare tire was wobbling down the ramp. The engine was still running. Quickly, we rolled the beetle back on its legs and climbed back in. The roof had been crushed down about a foot so the sprung doors no longer closed but protruded above the roof like the wings of a butterfly. We both held our respective door shut, and I steered with my right hand while Stan shifted with his left, driving around the transition road, down the off-ramp, and into the parking lot of the Pantry. We parked in a space out of view from the ramp or the street. At the time, it seemed like an exciting adventure, but looking back, we were beyond lucky. After this episode, my guardian angel applied for a transfer. By a miracle of good fortune, we were not caught. I was just twenty years old, underage for drinking, and even though the standard for intoxication was higher (0.10 percent), my blood alcohol almost certainly exceeded that at the time of the accident. Somehow, I managed to cheat death and avoid the societal penalties of my very poor judgment one more time.

I graduated from college a month later. Along with many of my classmates, I had developed a serious alcohol problem. I only drank on the weekends but consistently to moderate intoxication. Alcohol was the constant companion at all social occasions, and it was used to celebrate the highs of life and to mourn the lows. In the social environment of my college, alcohol was pervasive, and there were established rituals for experiencing both elation and sorrow, all of which involved getting drunk. Sadly, I never questioned the rationale. Was the alcohol to heighten the joy? Salve the grief? Obscure the pain? Erase the memory? It did none of those things, but it had become a strongly conditioned response to a wide variety of emotions.

Seattle (Associated Press)

PARENTS SUE FRATERNITY AFTER SON DIES AT PARTY

The parents of a University of Washington student who died in a fall at the Pi Kappa Phi house are suing the fraternity, saying he was encouraged to drink during a party game.

In the lawsuit filed this week in King County Superior Court, Don and Janice Jensen said that the May 2002 death of their 19-year-old son, Brett, followed a game called "Century Club" in which participants are supposed to drink a shot of beer every minute for 100 minutes.

(Author's note: If the shot glass was an ounce and a half, the participants would absorb nine ounces of alcohol in that period and have a blood alcohol of 0.25 percent at the end of the game. If the shot glass was two ounces, twelve ounces would be consumed, resulting in a blood alcohol of 0.35 percent).

5

FOR TEENS & YOUNG ADULTS

✦

Your Whole Life Changed in One Wasted Moment

The voice on the phone was sobbing.

"Mike, I'm pregnant. What are we going to do?"

You're numb. You can't believe what you just heard. The night it happened is a blurry memory. There was a party. Holly had been flirting with you all semester and that night she was coming on big-time. You both had more than a few beers. The next thing you knew, she had her hand in your pants and was leading you downstairs. You weren't prepared for this and had no condoms. You thought you had pulled out before orgasm but apparently not soon enough.

What are you going to tell your parents? What are you going to say to her parents?

One phone call and your life is changed forever. No more free time. No hanging with your friends. You need to support and care for a baby 24/7. You're going to have to work after school until graduation at a minimum wage job. Forget about going away to college. You'll be going to community college and it will take you twice as long to finish, if you ever do.

Your whole life changed in one wasted moment.

You thought Ty was going too fast but, what the hell, it was a fun ride! There are shrieks from the backseat and someone laughs as he throws a couple of empties out the window.

The curve is too sharp and Ty can't hold it. The car careens onto the right shoulder. Ty swings the wheel left and the car spins into the oncoming headlights.

The lights drive straight into your door, the passenger side. There is an explosion of glass and a sickening crunching of metal. An instant later, another explosion, and the smell of burning rubber. The crumbling frame pushes you toward Ty and the hood of the oncoming car folds up in front of you. There are muffled screams from the backseat. There is grinding and scraping and screaming. Then, nothing.

Ty's door is sprung and you both climb out around the air bags. There is sobbing from the backseat.

"Oh my God, my face." There is a huge laceration across Cody's forehead shaped like a trapdoor: something sharp had ripped back a huge piece of skin. Jagged and ugly, it is sitting on top of his head. There is blood everywhere. Patrick isn't moving.

There are screams from the other vehicle. Smoke is pouring from the crumbled engine compartment.

You run to the window. A woman is sobbing uncontrollably, rocking back and forth, cradling a man's head in her lap. Blood is pouring from his nose and eyes.

He will die in her arms.

For you and for Ty, the nightmare isn't over. It's just beginning. Vehicular manslaughter, DUI, minor in possession—the list seems endless and the sentence will be even longer. But it can't compare to the knowledge that your carelessness cost someone his life.

Your whole life changed in one wasted moment.

You've just left Dave's after a few beers. You're heading home, driving cautiously to avoid being pulled over. You try not to drink and drive, but you had no other ride home. Somebody's tailgating you, flashing his brights for you to speed up. You pull up at a signal. A pickup with two guys in it pulls up beside you at the light. The guy in the passenger seat gives you a dirty look, mouths "f____ you," and gives you the finger. You are pissed off; you're trying to drive cautiously and these guys are giving you grief, so you return the gesture. Before you know what's happening, they both jump out of their truck with baseball bats. Your window is broken in an instant; you can't get away quick enough. They drag you out of your car. They hit you repeatedly with the bats. White-hot pain sears your head, your back, and your arms. You are down, covering your head, and now they are kicking you, stomping you with their heavy boots. Then everything goes dark.

You awake in the county hospital. Your head is throbbing and it feels bigger than a watermelon. Your left arm is in a cast. Your nose is running briskly, dripping on your massively swollen upper lip. The drainage from your nose is cerebrospinal fluid leaking from a crack in the base of your fractured skull. The healing of the torn covering of the brain will put you at risk for seizures; you will need to take an antiseizure medication and will not be able to drive for two years. You are lucky to be alive.

Your whole life changed in one wasted moment.

You awoke that morning feeling a bit strange: a little achy. Halfway through algebra, you started feeling waves of chills alternated with fever, so you skipped volleyball practice after school and went straight home. By the time you arrived home you were feeling horrible. Every muscle in your body hurt, you had a splitting headache, and you were burning up. Your mother tried to make you drink fluids, but you just lay still in bed and didn't move. Everything hurt.

The pain and blisters in your vagina began on the second day. There was a burning, as though a torch had been placed up inside. Urinating was agony. You had to get into a lukewarm bath to void. Even then, it was painful.

After two days, you were not better. Your mother took you to the doctor. It didn't take long to make a diagnosis. One look at your vulva and the doctor said in an apologetic tone, "Sarah, this is Herpes Simplex, type II. This is a primary outbreak."

You were in shock. How could that be? There is only one boy, Tom, and he always used a condom. Then, you remembered that night after the basketball game. You had been drinking with some friends and Zack was sitting by you. He was cute and sexy, and you got very drunk. You may have passed out, but couldn't remember. You were pretty sure you had sex though because your panties were all wet and sticky when you came around.

Now this. What does it mean?

It means that for the rest of your life you will have recurrent painful outbreaks of blisters in your vagina: sometimes from sex, sometimes from stress, sometimes from periods. You'll be contagious, even when you don't have blisters, to anyone with whom you have sex. And if you get pregnant, you may transmit the infection to your new baby if delivering while broken out. In order to prevent the infection from causing severe brain damage to your newborn baby, a Caesarian section may be required.

You will experience a lifetime of pain and embarrassment.

One wasted moment and your life was changed forever.

His parents were in the waiting room. Someone would have to tell them. That someone would be you. You don't need to give them the gory details, that the bullet entered beneath the left eye, went through the maxillary sinus at an upward angle, entered the skull through the floor, tore through the meninges, and sliced into the base of the brain. You don't need to include that it compressed half the cerebral hemisphere against the skull as it exited, explosively ripping a three-inch piece of bone and skin off as it exited three inches behind the right ear.

It didn't matter now that his friend was just playing after they shared half a fifth of his parents' whiskey. It didn't matter that he thought the gun wasn't loaded.

All they need to know is that he died instantly. A bright flash and he was gone. No pain. No suffering. There was nothing that could be done once the gun fired.

But it won't be easy.

He was their only child.

And he was nine years old.

One wasted moment and a life was ended.

Every story in this chapter is true. Every one of the lives involved was irretrievably altered by alcohol. Alcohol caused a lapse in judgment, common sense, and motor skills, and consequences that would last a lifetime.

Have you ever held a belief that was so strong that you never doubted it? And then one day awoke to the realization that you had been completely wrong?

Maybe it was a friend that you confided in and trusted only to find out that she was sharing all your secrets with others. Maybe it was a lover who was unfaithful. Maybe it was a fact you learned in school that you thought was as solid as the law of gravity. Then one day you realized you had been mistaken all along.

Alcohol is like that. Everyone does it and it feels so good; it adds to the enjoyment of friends and occasions. But not everyone can drink occasionally and moderately. Have you experienced one of the following?

You realize that alcohol makes you angry and argumentative. You don't like it but you don't stop.

You realize that 99 percent of the confusion and screwups in your life are because of alcohol. But you don't stop.

You realize that your drinking friends are alcoholics. You look in the mirror and you realize you are too. But you don't stop.

In a moment of clarity, of honesty, or of humiliation, you come to a realization that many of the problems in your life are a result of drinking too much and too often. And you hate it. But you can't stop.

For young people it could be so simple. Just don't start. Twenty-five percent of alcoholics are teenagers (Student Affairs Handbook 2005–2006). If you have already started, stop before it's too late.

Before the unwanted pregnancy.

Before the vehicular manslaughter.

Before the DUI.

Before somebody beats your brains out in a brawl.

Before you contract a sexually transmitted disease that you will have the remainder of your life.

Before you are introduced to other addictive drugs that can enslave you.

Before you take a drug like meth that permanently changes your personality or thought process (Rumbaugh 1976).

Several of my recovering alcoholic friends had alcoholic fathers. Growing up, they vowed they would never be like their dads. And they knew they should never take that first drink. But wanting to be a part of the crowd, wanting to fit in, they did. And within a year or two, they were alcoholics as well.

Don't start. What seems like so much fun at first can lead to untold misery. Suicide is the third leading cause of death in teens (Morbidity and Mortality Weekly Report 2004, 471) and, in males, is on the rise (Morbidity and Mortality Weekly Report 2005, 377). Many are alcoholics on the fast track to hopelessness and helplessness. Depression that is so prevalent in teens is compounded by the depression of alcohol.

Remember: one wasted moment can change your whole life.

6

WE ARE KILLING OUR CHILDREN: ADVERTISING, THE MEDIA, AND THE BRAINWASHING OF AMERICA'S YOUTH

The handsome young cowboy flirted with the young ladies at the boarding barn. He sipped a beer and groomed his sleek chestnut quarter horse before putting him back in the stall. A small knot of horsewomen gathered at the wash rack smiled, giggled, and blushed at his simple attentions. Tall, lean, friendly, and a good horseman, the young man was liked by everyone at the barn. He was new at Cal Poly, was majoring in Ag Science, and had a bright future. He paused to visit with coeds and sipped another beer. Then he was in his truck and on his way home.

He never made it.

Driving out of town, he was going too fast for the curve on Foothill and rolled his truck. Without a seat belt, he was ejected from the truck and was airborne at fifty miles an hour; his head slammed into a brick wall at the entrance to a housing tract just beyond the curve. It nearly exploded from the impact. Mercifully, he was dead at the scene. Dead at twenty years of age. His blood alcohol was 0.15 percent. Everyone at the Horse Unit was stunned by the sudden loss.

You'll remember, when I was a senior in college, I had a frighteningly similar experience. A friend and I had seat belts on as my Volkswagen rolled and, unbelievably, I was unscathed. My friend scraped an elbow on the pavement as we rolled.

I knew that I had been fortunate, but as a young person used to risk taking, I didn't really realize how profoundly blessed I had been to survive the wreck, to escape life-altering physical injuries, to avoid killing my friend, and least of all, to avoid arrest. A felony drunk-driving conviction would prevent acceptance into medical school or licensure to practice when I graduated. With nearly forty years of hindsight, I truly believe it was God's hand that kept me safe that afternoon. I only wish I had learned from the experience sooner than I did and recognized my problem with alcohol for what it was. But I didn't. Instead, I just felt really lucky and became somewhat of a legend in the fraternity for my coolness under fire.

She was blonde and beautiful, and it was her twenty-first birthday. Cristal King promised her mother that she would not drive. After a night of celebration, she accepted a ride home from a twenty-three-year-old young man who had a prior DUI and was driving on a suspended driver's license. He was trying to impress her with the power and handling of his convertible sports car, but he misjudged the curve on the off-ramp, slamming the passenger side of the car into the retaining wall. The lovely young life in the seat beside him was instantly snuffed out. An only child, the pride of her loving and hardworking parents, was dead, her spectacular smile gone forever. The drunk driver didn't kill one person that night; he killed three. Her parents are dead emotionally and may never recover. I remember the haunted face of Cristal's mother at the trial. Robbed of her only child, she wanted harsh punishment for the driver. His blood alcohol was 0.10 percent, hardly enough to impair his driving ability but certainly enough to impair his judgment. Convicted of involuntary manslaughter and sentenced to prison, his life will never be the same. A banner hangs on the retaining wall where she died, reading "A Cristal clear reminder: Don't drink and drive." Her mother places bouquets of fresh flowers in a vase at the base of the wall in an attempt to keep her memory alive.

Two high school chums swigged a six-pack on a warm spring evening and decided to drive into town. The driver misjudged a curve and the vehicle slammed into a huge oak tree at the road's edge. The passenger died; the driver suffered massive chest injuries but survived to carry the physical and emotional scars of that night all his life. And incredibly, there were letters to the editor of the local paper the following week stating that the oak tree was a hazard and really needed to be removed.

When are we going to say *enough*?

A young mother was driving her two children to a soccer game. On the main street coming into town, she was hit head-on by a drunk young man passing on a two-lane road. One of the children was killed; the other spent a month in the hospital and months in rehabilitation. The drunk driver was unscathed physically but will see the faces of those children and the grief-crazed, tearstained face of the mother for the rest of his life.

Two young men with a twelve-pack of beer were out joyriding in a rural part of the county. The driver missed a curve, ran off the road, hit a power pole, and broke a fifteen-thousand-volt wire, which dangled just outside the door where the car came to rest. The driver may have recognized the danger if he were sober, but he certainly didn't drunk. He struggled out of the car, brushed the wire, and was instantly electrocuted. He was the oldest of three brothers, bright and handsome, captain of the football team, and headed to UC-Davis the next fall. His parents, his brothers, and his classmates were numb with shock.

How can we stop this?

An unsuspecting motorist was driving into town on Highway 1, slowing to fifty-five as he approached the first set of signals on the west side. Suddenly, a man walking beside the highway ran into his lane of traffic. The driver didn't even have time to hit the brakes. The pedestrian was dead on impact. The papers speculated that the dead man, a student at Cal Poly, had committed suicide. But he was doing well in school and his friends said he was not depressed. Two weeks later, a one-paragraph article reported that his blood alcohol was 0.34 percent.

He shouldn't have been able to stand up, let alone walk. Where were his friends? Who let him leave the party that drunk? Was he really trying to kill himself? We'll never know. The only certainties are his death and the shocking impact on the motorist who hit him.

I live in a county with a population of 225,000. The local papers reflect the small-town feeling by featuring county news in the front-page headlines. Articles on traffic deaths keep me constantly aware of the tragedies that alcohol has created for so many. Every year at least two of our high school students die in alcohol-related accidents. Often I know their families. The whole community mourns.

I feel a great sadness whenever I read about another needless death. I visualize the devastated parents, the shocked friends, and the guilt-ridden driver. And the scenario plays out over and over again. Only the actors are different.

I also experience anger. When is our society going to recognize the devastating effects of alcohol on our youth? How will we stop this hemorrhaging of the life-blood of our society, these beautiful young people who have a momentary, alcohol-induced loss of judgment?

The advertising industry and the news media aren't behind us. They have brainwashed three generations of young people with the sexiness of liquor.

It begins with kids in junior high and high school. All major sports events, the X Games, and popular television shows run beer commercials. And they are clever, sexy, and funny.

There are the extraordinarily attractive bikini-clad babes surrounding the guy who is drinking the right beer. Overt as well as subliminal messages that the right choice in beer will guarantee getting the girl, being cool with your friends, or enhancing your snowboarding skills are prevalent. For this pubescent audience, the importance of belonging to a peer group is paramount, as demonstrated by the popularity of baggy clothes, tattoos, and piercings. Advertisers understand peer identification and effectively use it to draft beer drinkers.

For the older age group, there are male-bonding scenes made all the more poignant with the right beer—like watching the big game with the "boys" and the right beer.

For the health conscious, there is the beer brewer sifting hops through his hand, ever so seriously explaining that beer is a "natural food" and emphasizing the importance of its freshness, which is why his company has breweries in every major city in the country.

For the patriotic, there's the magnificent beer wagon being pulled by the strongest, most beautiful draft horses imaginable. How can you not admire that? They have become cultural icons. Yet, what are they promoting?

Is there something disingenuous about a beer manufacturer promoting "responsible drinking"? Is that an oxymoron? And now, it's important to designate a driver, so everybody else in the group can drink more freely, consume more, and have a guilt-free drunk.

For the thirty something, upwardly mobile set, the delivery system for America's drug of choice is different. It is wine. It is incredible how the wine industry has grown in the last two decades. The association of sophistication with wine knowledge and appreciation has been one of the great marketing coups of the wine industry. Thirty years ago, the wine shelf in your local liquor store had one aisle of jug wines and a section of screw-top Tokays and ports for the itinerant wino crowd. Now, half the space in large liquor stores is devoted to thirty different wine varieties from fifty different wineries. Wine-tasting classes and wine clubs have developed in every small community, and better homes have temperature- and humidity-controlled wine cellars. What a remarkable advertising and promotional success!

Years ago, I was one of them. I swirled and swished and sniffed the wine of the week with the like-minded folks. And we talked about "legs" and "nose" and "body," and we waxed poetic about the aromas: "There's a subtle hint of clove here." "Do you detect a bit of mint?" "This wine has vegetable overtones." And we took copious notes and stored them away in our files. I can't deny that I enjoyed those evenings and that I learned a lot about wines and wine making. But I also can't deny that I have seen many of those wine club friends drunk a good portion of the time at those meetings and at the formal "wine dinners." Are we deluding ourselves? Is "wine education" just an excuse, a rationalization for getting drunk? It is, for many, exactly that. If you disagree, answer one question. If it's the aroma, the color, the body, and the subtle tastes that are really important, why not take the alcohol out? Nonalcoholic wines are available but unpopular. Wine drinkers want the alcohol. That's why they are drinking.

It was a brilliant coup for the wine industry when medical scientists published that one glass of red wine is good for the heart. What is often overlooked is that the study states "a glass," which is six or eight ounces of wine with dinner; I'm sure it is good for their heart. But people who drink only one glass of wine with dinner are as rare as smokers who smoke only one cigarette a day. For the high-functioning alcoholics of the world whose delivery system of choice is wine, that medical study legitimized their addiction.

In another remarkable advertising bonanza, the medical community published that "moderate alcohol intake" raises high-density lipoproteins or HDLs, the good fraction of cholesterol. But studies demonstrating that moderate alcohol consumption also increases one's risk of developing a number of cancers, including breast cancer, aren't made available to the public. The powerful alcohol industry filters the information.

Public relations and advertising firms have created a grand illusion about the wonder of drinking liquor. Be observant of the ads on television, billboards around town, or the displays at liquor stores and supermarkets. Notice how stacks of cases of beer are strategically placed where they intercept the most foot traffic. Observe the labels on the cartons celebrating whatever season we are in, because every season is a season to drink.

It is ironic that public opinion has swung so adamantly against cigarette smoking and the tobacco industry and yet still embraces fantasies about alcohol. Do you remember the old commercial for cigarettes produced during and after World War II? The star of the World Series is shown on a billboard, endorsing a brand of cigarette and claiming that it improved "his wind." The rugged Western star offers that his brand of smoke improves his appetite. And people bought it. In view of our present knowledge, these advertisements are ludicrous. Given the health facts of drinking alcohol, so are advertisements about liquor. We have simply traded one poison for another. And yet, the general public remains uneducated about the negative effects of alcohol. They lament a drunk wandering the streets and then are totally shocked when their annual routine blood test shows liver enzyme elevations from the three highballs they drank the night before their physical. They deplore the death toll from drunk drivers but are careful to drive the back roads home after a dinner party. They are mystified when they develop burning in their feet during their late sixties and the neurologist makes a diagnosis of "peripheral neuropathy," most often caused by chronic excessive alcohol intake.

I found it most interesting to learn that Philip Morris Corporation, a name made infamous in class action lawsuits for tobacco-related illness, owns Miller Brewing Company, producing some of the cleverest media campaigns ever for beer. The tobacco giant, fearing negative publicity from name recognition, asked its stockholders to approve a change to the Altria Group, an innocuous moniker for a mass killer who has simply changed weapons.

Motion pictures and television often glorify the world of intoxication rather than create an honest view of the risks of alcohol abuse. A trailer for a recent movie targeting the teen crowd chronicles a group of very cool snowboarders, and their excessive drinking is glorified. When one of the group passes out, they put him in his car, spin it around on the icy road, and then rouse him. He thinks he's really driving and panics while all his buddies fall down laughing. In another sequence, they all enormously enjoy watching a friend vomit as a result of excess drinking. With messages like these to our young people, how can we ever hope to bring home the real tragedy of alcoholism?

Another popular myth perpetuated by the movies is how well alcohol works as a tool of seduction. Every college-age male believes that after a couple of glasses of wine, the beautiful girl will succumb to his charm. And occasionally she does. The epidemic of sexually transmitted diseases and unwanted pregnancies is the result of the abandonment of good sense and reason produced by that same amount of alcohol, yet that message is seldom if ever presented.

Stemming the tide of popular opinion and changing the perception of three generations of alcohol users is an enormous task. But small victories are being won. Faced with the knowledge that graduation night is the most dangerous night of a teen's life, parents and educators have joined forces to organize "Sober

Grad Night," all-night celebrations where kids are closely supervised and a variety of fun activities are substituted for the former ofttimes drunken revels. New Year's Eve parties are being replaced by alcohol-free "First Night" celebrations in towns and cities nationwide. High schools have organized school-wide alcohol awareness campaigns where, in an assembly, the students view a mock-up of a drunk-driving collision. Emergency personnel minister to the "victims," who are students of the school. One dies and others are injured. The following day, the whole school attends the "funeral" and hears the parents and friends of the victim speak. Throughout the two days, an anonymous and silent representative of death appears in classrooms and removes students to represent the number of youth who are killed by alcohol each day.

It is an uphill battle. Creating an awareness of the physical, emotional, and spiritual damage that alcohol wreaks on our culture requires that we fight economic giants that reap huge revenues from the sale of alcohol. Wine grapes are the number one agricultural revenue for my county of residence. Sales of alcoholic beverages reach into the billions of dollars, and if the alcohol industry feels threatened by a changing public perception of their products, they will fight to maintain their markets.

Changes are possible, but we have to begin with the young. Once a pattern of alcohol abuse is established, it is very hard to alter. If we can keep kids from starting, however, we may be able to save a lot of lives. Perhaps a documentary revealing the tragic aspects of drinking could be required viewing for all high school students. If kids saw the devastation left in the wake of a drunk driver's path, watched an alcoholic die of ruptured esophageal varices, saw the mania of a violent drunk in lockup, heard the verbal abuse of a drunk spouse, or saw the bruises of a drunk-battered wife, maybe a few could say no. If we keep kids from starting, it would be a lot easier than getting them to quit. If someone had helped me question the "normalcy" of my parents' drinking as I was growing up, I might have seen my problem for what it was years ago. As I was, there are millions of young people at risk in this country today. It is worth a try to attempt to reach them.

We owe them that.

BOB HAYES

September 30, 2002

To the Editor:

Bob Hayes died last week. He was fifty-nine years old. He died of kidney failure due to complications from terminal cancer but, in reality, he had been dead for years. He was an alcoholic and addicted to cocaine.

Bob Hayes is the only man to own an Olympic gold medal and a Super Bowl ring. He was "the fastest human" for ten years. He won the Olympic gold medal in the 100-meter dash in the 1964 Tokyo Olympics and anchored the four-by-100-meter relay team, taking the baton eight yards behind two other competitors and annihilating them at the finish.

He was drafted by the Dallas Cowboys as a wide receiver, and he literally redefined the game. In those days, defensive backs could manhandle receivers, grabbing them, knocking them down even past the five yards from scrimmage that is the rule today. Problem was, they couldn't catch Bob Hayes to knock him down. He was so fast that one fake and he was past the defensive back and in the clear, awaiting Roger Staubach's perfect spiral.

He had good hands, surprising for a man hired purely for his speed. And he had good moves once he caught the ball, eluding many frustrated safeties in the open field. In his first three seasons, he caught forty-six touchdown passes, a record that stood for two decades. He is still third on the all-time list.

If you ever saw him in a track singlet and shorts, you would think you had seen the perfect human body. With massive thighs and chiseled muscles, he was beautiful to look at.

But, somewhere in the limelight of stardom, Bob Hayes found alcohol and cocaine. And they killed him. But before killing him, they ruined him. They reduced this most superb of human beings to a shell of his former self.

After fifteen years, losing battle after battle for sobriety, he finally got clean and sober, but the damage was done. I heard several interviews with him a few years before he died which reflected his brain impairment from the drugs and alcohol. His speech was permanently slurred, the thought processes infantile. It made me want to cry for this once magnificent warrior. But that's what alcohol and drugs will do. They will destroy a body and a mind. Worst of all, they corrupt the spirit. They did it to Bob Hayes.

We mourn him. We shake our heads and say "what a tragedy." But we as individuals and as a society do not acknowledge alcohol's potential for destruction. We glorify it. Coors has a new advertising theme: "Official Sponsor of Boys' Night Out." The images are of drunken revelry rife with implied sexual promiscuity. And that's cool. We are initiating a whole new generation of alcoholics. If they ever wake up to their addiction, they will have squandered two or three decades of their lives. If they are as unlucky as Bob Hayes, they may be permanently brain-impaired from drinking. They may lose their minds and their souls.

When are we going to recognize the magnitude of this problem?

7

ALCOHOL AND YOUR HEALTH: THE GREAT HOAX

It's not that you have been lied to; you've just been told a limited portion of the facts. The behemoth multinational corporations that market alcoholic beverages watch their stock prices soar every time a study is published demonstrating that alcohol is good for your health. And drinkers, many of whom are in denial that they have a problem or are in the early stage of alcoholism, can rationalize that their addiction is actually good for them.

Is it really?

Mark Twain is quoted as saying that there are three kinds of falsehood: "Lies, damn lies, and statistics." So it is with data presented by the popular media regarding alcohol. First, the alcohol corporations' spin doctors tell you only what they want you to know. Second, they have narrow and unrealistic definitions of terms that don't match the public perceptions of drinking.

Narrowly defined, "moderate alcohol consumption" lowers health risk from cardiovascular disease. But it raises risk for various cancers, hepatitis, osteoporosis, immune suppression, accidents, and suicide. That's the part they don't tell you.

But I will.

Let's start with a risk analysis of death at all stages of life. In youth, death rates are higher for accidents, suicide, homicide, and cancer than they are for heart disease. In middle age, the same is true, but cardiovascular disease is catching up. In old age, cardiovascular disease overtakes the other causes of death. Statistically, before the age of seventy-five, cancer and external causes of death are more common than heart disease. After seventy-five, heart disease becomes more important. Put simply, if we don't die of cancer, sooner or later our heart is going to give out.

With that background, let's examine the health risks of alcohol and carefully analyze the statistics and definitions used to perpetrate the great hoax that drinking alcohol is good for you.

ALCOHOL AND CANCER

John was a strikingly handsome man when I first met him. He was in his early sixties, was tall and lean, and had thick black hair silvered at the temples, a warm smile, and a large hand with a firm but friendly handshake. But John had a perplexing problem: an unusual and difficult-to-treat form of oral cancer. Two years prior, his dentist had noticed an ominous-looking white patch on the inside of his left cheek. An oral surgeon had done a biopsy. The diagnosis was "squamous cell carcinoma in situ."

The term "in situ," literally translated "in place," is a concept that needs some explaining. When cancer begins in the skin (or the mouth equivalent, the mucous membrane), it begins in the top or cellular layer called the epidermis or mucosa, respectively. Here, cancer cells may first arise through mutation, divide, and grow into a colony of malignant cells. They are confined to the top layer, however, biologically fenced out by a tough little membrane beneath the epidermis/submucosa called the basement membrane. Before these cancer cells can invade into the deeper tissues, a new mutation has to occur in one of the cancer cells that produces an enzyme which can eat a hole in the basement membrane and allow the cells to invade. Without this enzyme, the cells are confined to the top layer and can grow for an indefinite period of time, "in situ." Thus, although imminently dangerous, such a proliferation of cells is "precancerous."

So, John had this patch on the inside of his cheek that showed in situ cancer. John's was squamous cell, a term that describes the flat platelike cells of the upper epidermis or mucosa. Because, most commonly, the cancer cells developing in any area of the body arise from normal cells that belong there, squamous cell cancer is the most common malignancy of the mouth. The word "carcinoma" is a Greek word that is synonymous with "cancer." They both mean "crab" and describe the gross appearance of a cancer as it spreads out into the tissues. The roots grossly resemble legs or claws invading into normal tissue from the main body of the cancer.

There are three main risk factors for squamous cell carcinoma of the mouth: tobacco, alcohol, and poor oral hygiene. Surprisingly, John only had one factor: alcohol. He owned a very prestigious winery in our area and was a noted authority on wine. John never smoked and his dental care was impeccable.

So, how did he develop oral cancer?

Because alcohol alone can cause it.

John had his carcinoma excised but it wasn't three months after the sutures were removed that several new patches developed, one at the edge of the surgical scar and one on the inside of the other cheek. They both showed carcinoma in situ. Unfortunately, this is a common occurrence with oral cancer, as it is a multifocal disease. The negative influence that created the first cancer affected many other oral mucosal cells as well, and distinctly new lesions continue to arise.

It was remarkable that John had no other risk factors than his wine drinking. And he was light-years away from being an alcoholic. But he tasted, sampled, and evaluated a lot of wine. At large tastings, he might sample two dozen wines. After evaluating the "nose" or fragrance, he would sip a small amount of a wine, swish it around, draw a small amount of air into his mouth, and experience the full flavor of the wine. By using this method of tasting, the wine spent a great deal more time in the mouth than if he were just drinking it.

John went to Stanford, where his cancers were excised and a large graft was placed on the inside of his cheek to cover the defect. As the graft healed, it contracted, shrinking his cheek down so that he could barely open his mouth. On one of our follow-up visits, I could not insert a tongue depressor sideways between his teeth. I injected some steroid in the scar and it loosened up enough to admit the tongue depressor, but just barely.

John's surgery was followed by radiation, five days a week for seven weeks. His mouth grew so raw that he required a feeding tube to take nutrition. Two months after his final radiation treatment, two new patches were noted on the right cheek. Both were positive for cancer and one was frankly invasive. Despite its removal, the cancer had spread to the lymph nodes beneath his jaw within six months. Radical neck surgery removed the nodes and some of the muscles of the right neck. Another course of radiation and chemotherapy produced a six-month remission, but a chest X-ray revealed several lung metastases, and severe hip pain led to a diagnosis of bony metastases in the pelvis. Within a year, John was dead. The widespread metastatic disease caused by squamous cell carcinoma was initiated by drinking wine.

John's cancer was uncommon, but the wine had to have played a role. He had no other risk factors, and as we will show later, alcohol is converted into cancer-causing acetaldehyde by bacteria in the mouth.

Although there are some back-page press reports and unobtrusive labeling of alcoholic beverages, the general public is not really aware that alcohol increases cancer risk. For a number of cancers, it does. Those cancers include the mouth, throat, esophagus, stomach, breast, liver, rectum, possibly the colon, and probably the pancreas. Interestingly, alcohol itself is not carcinogenic. You can bathe cells in tissue culture with alcohol and it does not produce cancerous cells. You can feed alcohol to a bacterium called *E. coli,* as is done with other substances in a well-known cancer screening called the Ames test, and it will not produce mutations. But if you take the first metabolic breakdown product of alcohol, a substance called acetaldehyde, and incubate it with tissue culture cells or feed it to *E. coli,* it will produce cancer cells. So it appears that acetaldehyde is one of the culprits in alcohol's role as a cancer-causing drug.

It has been shown that bacteria in the mouth, in the stomach, and throughout the gastrointestinal tract are capable of producing acetaldehyde from alcohol. The acetaldehyde then bathes the epithelial cells, presumably creating mutations and producing the cancerous changes. Everyone who drinks alcohol presumably has increased amounts of acetaldehyde in their saliva, stomach secretions, and bowel. Why then, doesn't everyone develop cancer? It appears that a genetic predisposition creates a wide variability among people in their ability to detoxify acetaldehyde. There is also a tremendous variability in how individual cells resist damage by acetaldehyde or repair the damage once it is done. The immune system also plays a key role in destroying cancer cells when they are at the one- and two-cell stage.

The liver also produces acetaldehyde from alcohol that then circulates in the bloodstream throughout the body. So all the tissues are exposed to this carcinogen, but not at the high concentrations produced in the gut by bacteria. It's a wonder then that alcohol is not associated with increased cancer risks in all organs of the body. There are, however, some surprising facts about alcohol's role in tumor formation elsewhere in the body.

Helen was a middle-aged housewife with three grown children. She did not meet the definition of an alcoholic, but she and her husband regularly shared a glass (or more) of wine with dinner, and she drank a bit more at weekend parties. Her gynecologist felt a breast lump on a routine exam in spite of the fact that she had a normal mammogram ten months prior. A biopsy showed intraductal carcinoma. Excision of lymph nodes revealed that three of twelve nodes had microscopic spread of the tumor. She underwent radiation therapy and chemotherapy and has been on Tamoxifen for over three years now. To date, there is no evidence of recurrence of her breast cancer.

Helen had no family history of breast cancer. She had none of the other known risk factors for breast cancer such as early onset of menstruation, having no children, having children later in life, failure to breast-feed, or hormone replacement therapy. She had three children in her twenties, breast-fed them all, and declined hormones after menopause. But, she did drink alcohol regularly.

Could that have played a role in developing breast cancer?

Surprisingly, yes. Several studies have shown an increase in breast cancer associated with alcohol intake. And these were not "heavy" drinkers. One study showed that women who drank one glass of wine a day had a 30 percent increase in breast cancer over a group that did not drink at all. The mechanism is not known, but perhaps breast tissue is more sensitive to the oncogenic ("onco" meaning "cancer," "genic" meaning "to give rise to") effects of acetaldehyde.

In the recent past, reports that a specific hormone replacement therapy (Prempro) may slightly increase a woman's risk of breast cancer have caused a huge furor in the press. Millions of women have given up hormone replacement and face the risk of osteoporosis, atrophy (thinning) and increased sensitivity of vaginal tissue, and heart disease due to a seriously flawed study (according to my obstetrician-gynecologist friends). Concurrently, there is solid evidence that alcohol definitely increases the risk of breast cancer, yet you don't see these same women giving up their wine because they are unaware of alcohol's potential danger.

Breast cancer is on the increase, especially in First World countries. Could it be partially due to an increase in alcohol consumption in women?

Yes, probably. In a startling recent study, it was found that women in upscale and affluent Marin County north of San Francisco have a 9 percent higher incidence of breast cancer than women in twenty-four other counties examined. In addition, the rate of breast cancer was increasing 3.6 percent per year, *six times higher* than the national average. Looking at all the possible variables that may have contributed to the increase, researchers found that women who developed breast cancer were more likely to consume two or more drinks per day than were women in a control group who did not develop breast cancer.

So perhaps alcohol isn't so good for your health after all. But that's not what you hear from the wine marketers. They would have you think it is good for your health. If you are talking exclusively about cardiovascular health, it is. However, if you are talking about death from other causes, it is not.

Bill was mid-fifties, the picture of health. Lean and tan, he played on a basketball team in the local recreation league. He sold insurance and was quite successful. He was a moderate to heavy drinker: two glasses of wine with dinner, a margarita and wine with dinner at weekend parties and during meals with clients. His only medical issue was a nagging problem with hemorrhoids since his late twenties. He had undergone two previous surgeries, so when he developed new rectal bleeding, he just assumed it was another hemorrhoid. The bleeding wasn't too severe and the memory of the painful removal was vivid. Bill would wait until the pain and bleeding were really disruptive before he would subject himself to another surgery.

When he had to wear diapers to keep from ruining his pants, he figured it was time. But he and his wife had booked a cruise to celebrate their twenty-fifth anniversary, so he postponed his doctor's appointment. He knew the proctologist personally from the country club and wasn't looking forward to the jokes in the locker room and the surgeon's rough technique. So his appointment was delayed another couple of months.

Lying on the table, naked, draped with a sheet, Bill felt embarrassed and incredibly vulnerable. He silently cursed his mother's side of the family, all of whom had hemorrhoids at a young age.

Dr. Schultz's brusqueness left little room for tact or empathy. He groped around for a brief moment and then straightened up.

"This isn't any hemorrhoid. This is a tumor."

And it was.

Rectal cancer.

Schultz did a biopsy and left a shocked patient to dress in silence and fear. The biopsy showed rectal cancer, a tumor the size of a Ping-Pong ball. There was a flurry of tests. A CT scan showed spread to the nodes of the pelvis.

Within a week, Bill had surgery. The tumor, the rectum, and the distal colon were removed. A colostomy was done, followed by two months of radiation and a year of chemotherapy. Despite aggressive measures, nodules of the tumor appeared in the liver and then in the lung. A different chemotherapy was tried to no avail. As Bill's liver filled with metastatic nodules, there was less healthy liver functioning to detoxify the ammonia and other toxins produced by normal metabolism. Bill slowly slipped into hepatic coma and died.

He was fifty-six.

Was Bill's cancer caused by alcohol? Alcohol contributed. Studies reveal that there is an increase in rectal cancer in moderate to heavy drinkers. That is due in part to the acetaldehyde at work again on the cells of the rectal mucosa. There are other factors as well, including a high-fat diet.

Not only does alcohol contribute to the development of cancers in many areas of the body, but once a cancer has become established, no matter where it arose, there is evidence that spread of that cancer may be facilitated by alcohol. The spread of a cancer from the primary site to new areas, both adjacent to and at distant sites from the primary, is known as metastasis ("meta" meaning "change" and "stasis" meaning "place"). There are many factors that affect the ability of a tumor to metastasize; however, an important factor preventing such spread is a specialized immune cell, part of the T lymphocyte population called "natural killer T cells." These cells are like policemen patrolling your bloodstream and other tissues looking for trouble, searching for viruses, bacteria, fungi, yeast, and tumor cells. These cells are unique because they do not require previous immunization to a particular protein on the surface of a bacteria or tumor cell to work, and they are not specific for tumor or bacteria. They just attack anything that does not have the genetic profile of the host. These natural killer T cells, or "NK cells" as they are known, are extremely important in preventing metastasis. They patrol the body and attack and kill tumor cells spreading through the blood vessels and the lymph system.

Alcohol suppresses the number of functioning NK cells in the body, promoting the spread of cancer to distant sites.

In a study using mice and experimental melanoma cells, mice with blood alcohol levels in the range of moderate to heavy alcohol use had a 50 percent depletion of NK cells and an increase in metastases to the lung. As an aside, sunburn has also been shown to drastically reduce NK cell numbers, while vigorous exercise has been shown to increase NK cell numbers.

So, alcohol not only helps produce some cancers but also promotes their spread. Not surprisingly, these facts are not publicized. The alcohol industry, a powerful lobby, would highly discourage the publication of this information. Unfortunately, the medical field has failed you as well. I know of no oncologists who advise their patients to abstain from alcohol once they have been diagnosed with cancer. I do.

My friend, Scott, developed squamous cell carcinoma, metastatic to his neck, twelve years after he quit smoking and drinking heavily. In spite of aggressive surgery, radiation, and chemo, he lost a valiant battle.

Having watched Scott suffer, I find it hard to read and listen to the propaganda about moderate alcohol being healthy.

Carla felt as if she had the flu. She woke up in the morning nauseated and with a cramping pain in her belly. There was no fever but she couldn't keep anything down. When her symptoms lasted a week, she finally went to the doctor. He ran some tests and called her the next day, a note of concern in his voice. He ordered a CT scan for the following morning. The scan showed a large tumor in the pancreas. It was inoperable. Carla got a second opinion at City of Hope, but they concurred. Chemotherapy was a possibility, but they were pessimistic about the chances for success.

Miraculously, Carla's pancreatic cancer responded to chemotherapy. At this writing, she is well with a small but persistent tumor still present.

Pancreatic carcinoma is a leading cause of cancer-related deaths in this country. A direct link with alcohol consumption has not yet been established, although there is some strong incriminating evidence. Pancreatic cancers commonly have a peculiar gene rearrangement in a gene called K-ras. Such K-ras mutations have been correlated with alcohol consumption.

In addition to the cancer-causing properties of acetaldehyde, the promotion of metastases due to the decrease in natural killer (NK) T cells, and K-ras mutations, alcohol contributes to the development of cancers in another important way. There is a very important enzyme in many cells of the body, most importantly in the liver, called cytochrome p450. This enzyme is critical for the metabolism or processing of many substances in the body, especially breaking down drugs and detoxifying a variety of substances entering the body from the external environment. Alcohol induces a special variant of p450 called CYP 2E1, which, instead of detoxifying these chemicals, is responsible for changing some of them into carcinogens, thus producing a chemical environment conducive to the development of cancer. A number of substances known as pro-carcinogens are metabolized into carcinogens by CYP 2E1, and since alcohol increases the production of CYP 2E1, it results in higher concentrations of carcinogens as well.

In reviewing the medical literature on the health effects of alcohol, I found a Japanese study showing that drinkers died of all known forms of cancer more commonly than nondrinkers. Did you ever read that headline in your local newspaper? Hear it on the news?

When a study demonstrating a health benefit of alcohol is published, it makes the front page. When a study proving that alcohol is a carcinogen is published, it is buried on the back pages, if it appears at all.

Twenty-five years ago, the health hazards of tobacco were just being defined and the tobacco companies denied each new revelation. Now it is accepted fact that tobacco use is a serious health risk. The same is now becoming apparent with alcohol: there are serious cancer risks associated with its use. How long will it be before these facts are disseminated to the public, and the marketers of this toxic substance own up to its cancer-causing potential?

If you are afraid of developing cancer and dying of it, you should not drink!

If you have had cancer and you are afraid of a recurrence or metastasis, you should not drink!

ALCOHOL AND OSTEOPOROSIS

Gladys was walking down the back stairs with an armload of newspapers on the way to her garage. She missed the second step and fell, landing hard: buttocks on concrete. There was a blinding pain in her low back, as if she had been slashed with a sword. She sat there for nearly an hour, paralyzed with pain, before her husband, Harold, came looking for her. He called 911 and Gladys was whisked to the emergency room of the local hospital. The attending physician immediately suspected the problem, as he had seen two similar cases in senior women that week. A back X-ray confirmed his diagnosis. Gladys had a compression fracture of her second lumbar vertebra. She had broken her back.

Gladys was suffering from osteoporosis (osteo = bone, porosis = spongy), an epidemic disease of seniors, particularly women. Insidious in its development, osteoporosis is caused by a loss or resorption of calcium from skeletal bone. As the result of the hard fall, the weight of her upper body literally collapsed a weakened second lumbar vertebra. An almost cube-like vertebral body that was originally two and a half inches thick was now a little over an inch thick, causing severe pain (an eight or nine on the ten scale) that would last for several months.

Over the last fifteen years, I have watched my father become more and more stooped over. Now, in his mid-eighties, he is so hunched in the upper back region that he is perpetually looking at the ground. It is not possible for him to straighten up, nor can he turn from side to side. He is literally a hunchback, with a male equivalent of the "dowager's hump" so commonly seen in women. The hump, caused by osteoporosis, results from demineralized bone shrinking and remodeling. The front of the vertebra is thinner than the back, producing a forward bend. With time, the disc spaces between the vertebrae can be obliterated, and the vertebrae actually fuse.

As I watched this occur in my father, I was surprised by its severity and progression and mystified as to its cause. My dad had been a heavy smoker, one recognized cause of osteoporosis, but I knew lots of male smokers who didn't have the degree of osteoporosis seen in my dad. Although medium in height, he was a large-boned, muscular man—the last person in whom you would expect osteoporosis.

Then, as I researched the health effects of alcohol, I came across a reference in the literature that astonished me. Alcohol is a leading cause of osteoporosis. My dad's heavy drinking and smoking created an osteoporosis double whammy.

The baby boomer generation now approaching late middle age is a fertile ground for the development of osteoporosis. 40 percent of women in their fifties have osteopenia, a decreased level of calcium in the bone that is an intermediate step to osteoporosis, and the estimates are that fully half of adult women in America develop osteoporosis in their lifetime. The critical skeletal areas affected by osteoporosis are the vertebrae and the hip. The head of the femur, a large ball-like bone that fits into the hip socket, is connected to the vertical shaft of the femur by a relatively narrow bone called the neck that attaches at almost a right angle. It is here that the hip typically fractures, through an osteoporotic neck of the femur.

It certainly came as a surprise to me, an MD, that alcohol was a leading cause of osteoporosis. It is not common knowledge in the general population, let alone in the medical community. With all the information about diet, exercise, and hormone replacement in the press and self-help magazines, one would think somewhere there might be a mention of alcohol's contribution to this ubiquitous disease of the elderly.

Alcohol causes osteoporosis by lowering the amount of calcium in the bloodstream via two mechanisms. First, alcohol is a diuretic, increasing urine production by the kidney. Calcium and magnesium are passively carried out with the increased urine flow. Second, ingestion of alcohol decreases the production of parathyroid hormone. This hormone, produced by several pea-sized glands located adjacent to ("para") the thyroid gland, causes calcium levels to rise in the blood by increasing absorption from the gut and decreasing kidney excretion of calcium. When alcohol is ingested, the calcium level in the blood drops and the urinary excretion of calcium increases. These changes are maximized eight to twelve hours after intake. That means that people who drink on a daily basis are chronically depriving their bones of calcium.

Does alcohol consumption in the elderly account in part for the increase in osteoporosis and its morbidity?

Absolutely!

ALCOHOL AND THE IMMUNE SYSTEM

Helen was a former Army nurse. She drank bourbon straight up, every night, and didn't care who knew it. She was as tough as an old shoe, ran her ward at LA

County like her Army hospital, and didn't take any guff from anybody, especially any smart-ass intern. I liked her immediately. With Helen, there were no pretenses. And she liked me because I treated her with the deference she deserved after thirty years of nursing. Conversely, she made life miserable for one member of my internship team, an arrogant young doctor named Rob Heller. The son of a doctor, a silver spooner, Rob belittled the nurses and always insisted on being called "Doctor" Heller.

Helen had seen his type and his problem before. He had a severe case of chronic self-importantism. And she had the cure. She would wait until he had just settled into his bunk in the sleeping room to call him for a problem patient who hadn't had a bowel movement in three days. Then, "Doctor" Heller would have to get up, put on a glove, and "de-impact" the poor old lady, removing concrete-like nodules of stool from her rectum. By contrast, Helen would always let me know when the IV on one of my patients was causing problems so I could retape it or flush it out before it was useless. With Dr. Heller, she waited until the IV had infiltrated or was hopelessly plugged and then told him, necessitating its replacement.

Helen was a piece of work! In a month on her service, I'll bet Rob didn't get more than twenty minutes of sleep the nights that we were on call.

But Helen always seemed to be sick. Coughing, wheezing, and blowing her nose every five minutes, she carried one of those small packages of Kleenex in her coat pocket and replenished it two or three times a night from a large carton in her desk drawer. Helen caught every cold that came onto the wards. Since she had been exposed to illness and disease her entire career, one would think she'd be immune to every virus on earth, but the opposite was true.

Only years later did it make sense to me. It was the whiskey. Alcohol suppresses the immune system. Upper respiratory viruses are foreign invaders. When they reach the nasal passages or throat, they are supposed to be met by a small army of immune defenders. The virus may be confronted by a Langerhans cell, a modified histiocyte, which interacts with the virus, recognizing foreign proteins on its surface and presenting them to T lymphocytes. T lymphocytes, once activated, give off complex and sophisticated chemical messages that recruit other immune cells and, eventually, in about ten to fourteen days, produce antibodies that neutralize the invading virus. This takes time, and meanwhile, the virus is replicating and causing the host to be sick.

There is another platoon of the immune army that doesn't need time to fight back. Natural killer T cells (NK cells) nonspecifically attack any non-host proteins, whether they be on viruses, bacteria, fungus, or tumor cells. They may completely inactivate invading viral particles and prevent an infection, even before the more robust but delayed immune system gets into the act.

There is a catch. A number of physical stimuli influence the number and vigor of NK cells. Vigorous exercise has been shown, for instance, to increase the number of NK cells, yet alcohol decreases them significantly. That means that viruses attacking the host have time to multiply before the delayed system can muster the troops. The patient becomes ill.

So, no wonder Helen was always sick. The liquor did it to her. By decreasing the number of natural killer T cells, Helen was made more vulnerable to every virus that was coughed across her desk. And even more importantly, those same natural killer T cells are one of our most important defenders against cancer, probably destroying mutant cells before they have a chance to develop into significant tumors. So, not only was Helen sick all the time, but she bore a higher risk of developing cancer as well.

ALCOHOL MAKES ALLERGIES WORSE

Ron lives with two inhalers as constant companions. He has had asthma since he was a young child and it has, at times, been severe and unrelenting. In spite of that, Ron excelled as a high school and college cross-country runner and as a horseman, and he is a fine golfer. In recent years, however, the asthma has worsened, making him even more dependent on his inhalers and several pills that he takes to lessen the symptoms. He has experienced a lot of work stress as he climbs his way up the corporate ladder, and I always attributed his worsening to that. Imagine my surprise when, in the course of my research on the health effects of alcohol, I discovered that alcohol greatly aggravates allergies of all kinds, including asthma.

Allergies are a major cause of discomfort and disability for over a third of the population. They manifest as asthma, hay fever, eczema, and food allergies. Recent studies indicate that allergies are on the rise in the United States.

An abnormal antibody, present only in people with allergies, causes these diseases. The antibody is called IgE or immunoglobulin E. IgE does not occur in normal, nonallergic people unless they are infested with parasites, such as intestinal worms. There is some evidence that IgE may help defend against and destroy such parasites, but when they are gone the IgE levels drop to a negligible level. In allergic people, however, the IgE levels are almost always high. They are specifically developed against certain substances, known as allergens, like grass pollen in the case of hay fever, or peanuts in the case of food allergies. Allergists actually test patients for specific allergies by assaying the level of IgE in their blood that reacts to these substances, known as allergens.

The immune system, even when it malfunctions, is a marvel. Each individual IgE molecule is specific for a unique allergen. The IgE molecule for peanuts will not respond to the protein allergen in almonds, pecans, or any other nuts. That is because the specific molecule of IgE has a receptor on its surface that is composed of a series of amino acids that is unique to that allergen. The receptor, extending out from the surface of the IgE molecule, is like a trailer hitch; it will only fit a similar hitch on the trailer. The receptor has to be just the right size and shape to attach to the allergen. When the correct allergen is present, the receptor and allergen fit together like a lock and key or the cup and ball of the trailer hitch. Once the receptor docks with the allergen, the fused proteins react with a feisty little cell known as a mast cell, present throughout the body, to produce allergy symptoms. The aroused mast cell releases small granules stored within it that contain proteins which produce intense inflammation. Notable among these are histamine, bradykinin, and a pesky little protein called slow-reacting substance of anaphylaxis. Histamine causes intense itching, redness and swelling of the skin, and a spasm of the tiny muscles that encircle the airways in the lungs, causing the narrowing or constriction of the bronchioles so characteristic of asthma.

Most of our treatments for these allergic problems target the histamine and other mediators of inflammation. We treat itching with antihistamines and the swelling and inflammation of eczema and asthma with cortisone-like steroids that diminish the inflammation. But we are treating the results of the abnormal reaction after it happens, slamming the barn door after the horse is long gone. Our therapeutic efforts need to be focused on decreasing IgE production or blocking its reaction with the allergen. The latter is currently being developed. In Europe, proteins called "blocking antibodies" are being used which attach to IgE molecules and prevent them from seeking out their allergen. Chronic hives are being treated with some success by this strategy, and the future looks bright for this kind of treatment.

Reducing IgE is also an excellent rationale for diminishing allergic illness. Since one of the potent stimulants to IgE production is alcohol, abstaining from drinking should greatly reduce allergic symptoms in susceptible individuals. Speaking from personal experience, it does. I have one-tenth the sneezing and itchy, watery eyes in the spring than I had before I quit drinking. Part of that is attributable to eliminating alcohol. The rest is due to my intake of large doses of vitamin E, which has also been shown to decrease IgE production. Additionally,

IgE has a life span of ninety days in the bloodstream, so it requires a long-term commitment to realize a reduction of allergic symptoms.

Have you ever heard that alcohol increases allergy problems? Probably not. The conspiracy of silence by alcohol producers publicizes only the health benefits of alcohol, not the legion of illnesses and malignancies promoted by its use.

Allergic disease is on the increase in the United States. Is it, in part, because there is an increase in drinking?

Draw your own conclusion.

ALCOHOL AND GERD

Wayne thought he was dying. Sweat poured off his forehead as pain gripped him, deep in the middle of his chest. He couldn't lie down. This was the third time this week, and the nitroglycerin failed to help. He couldn't get his breath. Certain that he was having a heart attack, he called 911. The paramedics were there within five minutes. Everything was a blur. Almost instantly, they had put an oxygen mask over his face, taken his blood pressure and pulse, hooked him up to an electrocardiogram telemetry system, started an IV, and placed him on a gurney and into their unit. Code 3 to Mar Vista Hospital. There, after three hours of cardiac monitoring, blood tests to assay heart muscle damage, morphine, and oxygen, the emergency room staff concluded that it was not a heart attack. Rather, it was pain coming from the upper esophagus, badly irritated by acid contents that leaked back from a faulty valve at the opening to the stomach.

Previously called heartburn, a fairly accurate description, the condition is now referred to as gastroesophageal reflux disease, or GERD for short. It is common and on the increase.

Wayne has GERD. The corrosive contents of his stomach, rife with enzymes powerful enough to autodigest his own tissues and hydrochloric acid strong enough to dissolve the toughest gristle on a porterhouse steak, leak back into the esophagus and burn it. The mucosa or lining of the esophagus wasn't designed to withstand that chemical insult. The burn results in erosion of the mucosa, exposing the delicate collagen of the submucosa and the smooth muscle beneath it. Just like an acid burn on the skin, it heals with scarring and, with repeated episodes, the scarring infiltrates and replaces the muscle. The complex and precise process of peristalsis, where bands of smooth muscle encircling the esophagus gently milk food downward from mouth to stomach, is permanently impaired. The lower end of the esophagus becomes atonic (unmoving) and the essential muscular valve separating the esophagus from the stomach known as the cardio-esophageal sphincter is destroyed. The process gradually worsens, resulting in a scarred and rigid esophagus that doesn't function at all.

The enormous popularity of drugs that decrease stomach acid production is testimony to the widespread occurrence of GERD. These drugs are advertised heavily on television, an interesting twist on the marketing strategy of pharmaceutical companies: don't advertise to the doctors; advertise to the patients and they will solicit the drug from their physician.

Wayne has to wait a minimum of two hours after eating before he can lie supine, enough time to allow the stomach to fully empty so that there are no corrosive contents to backflow into the esophagus. He is not alone. There are millions of Americans with GERD who rationalize that it is the stress of the modern world, the odd hours that stressful lives create, and the bizarre eating schedules that are necessitated by unusual work schedules that increases the acid production in their stomachs. Doctors' orders to restrict their drinking go unheeded. They continue to consume the highball after work and the two or three glasses of wine with dinner followed by Prevacid or Tagamet. They eat and drink it all, then pop the "fix it" pill.

GERD is caused, in large part, by alcohol. Alcohol causes a relaxation of the cardio-esophageal sphincter that allows the acid contents of the stomach to reflux into the lower esophagus and burn it. Alcohol also impairs the motility or muscle action of esophageal peristalsis. The combination of drinking alcohol and lying down with a stomach full of food, acid, and digestive enzymes is the formula for creating GERD.

Wayne is happy now. He takes his Prevacid regularly ("Wow, Doc, is that stuff expensive!") so that he can eat and drink anything he wants without trips to the emergency room. Pharmaceutical companies are profiting, and we continue, for the most part, to be unaware of alcohol's role in the GERD epidemic.

ALCOHOL AND PERIPHERAL NEUROPATHY

Florence's muscular body and a quick mind belie her eighty-two years of age. She plays golf twice a week and volunteers at the hospital. But she complains bitterly of a burning sensation in her feet that is steadily worsening, comparable to walking on a bed of hot coals.

Florence suffers from peripheral neuropathy. The sensory nerves to the skin of her feet are damaged. Like wires with frayed insulation, the electrical messages carried in these nerves frequently short-circuit, causing the nerves to report abnormal sensations or feelings that aren't really there. The result is a combination of numbness, tingling, or burning that occurs in the lower legs and feet, especially on the soles. Present all the time, it is most distressing at night when many other sensory stimuli diminish. What had been slightly annoying warmth on the bottoms of the feet during the day becomes an intolerable searing pain at night. Unfortunately, this is an increasingly common problem for our senior population.

Three major causes of peripheral neuropathy are diabetes, nutritional deficiencies, and alcohol consumption. Oftentimes, there is no identifiable cause and it is written off as aging nerves. Many of these cases are probably caused by alcohol but the investigating doctor is not getting an adequate idea of how much the patient drinks, or used to drink, as many alcoholic patients lie about their habit.

Alcohol causes nerve damage by at least two mechanisms. First and foremost, it is a cell poison, damaging and killing nerve cells in the brain and spinal cord. With the death of peripheral nerve cells or neurons, there is a decreased sensation in the involved areas. If the nerves are damaged, they function abnormally and may report back peculiar sensations such as itching, tingling, or burning.

Alcohol also produces nerve damage as it may cause a deficiency of several vitamins that are essential for neuronal function. People who drink heavily often do not pay attention to eating well. Alcoholic calories take the place of good nutrition. When a person is intoxicated on a regular basis, he may not include the major food groups in every meal. For some heavy drinkers, the three major food groups may be beer, wine, and whiskey. The result is that foods with critical vitamins for healthy nerve function may be omitted.

Folic acid, thiamine (B_1), and vitamin B_{12} are thought to be critical for healthy nerve function. Not surprisingly, many alcoholics show low levels of these vitamins in their bodies and their neuropathies are indistinguishable from those produced by these deficiencies.

With an aging population, peripheral neuropathy is becoming more of a health problem. Many cases due to neuronal degeneration related simply to the aging process may not be preventable with our current medical knowledge. But many cases related to the chronic abuse of alcohol are.

We need to get the word out.

INSOMNIA

Brenda hasn't had a good night's sleep in twenty years. She attributes it to the stress of her work as a legal secretary for a very demanding boss and raising two boys as a single parent. Sleep deprivation adds to the stress, shortening her fuse with her kids and coworkers.

Brenda falls asleep promptly when retiring and sleeps soundly for four hours. Then she awakens, tossing and turning, thinking about the bills, her ex-husband's delinquency with the child support, and the contracts she prepared for her boss that day. She doesn't sleep the rest of the night. She would never suspect that it might be the two glasses of wine she has before and during dinner to relax.

Alcohol depresses nerve function, both in the brain and throughout the nervous system. This alcohol, although a relatively small amount, is enough to alter the delicate chemical balance in the brain. With the depression of nerve function, the alcohol produces a mild sedative effect, and the initiation of sleep comes easily. But when the three to five ounces of alcohol are completely metabolized (the liver can metabolize one to one and a half ounces per hour), there is a rebound hyperactivity of the nerves. This produces wakefulness and persists long enough to ruin a good night's sleep.

Alcohol also reduces rapid eye movement (REM) sleep, a stage of sleep associated with dreaming, thought to be important for resting and recharging one's emotional energy. Many regular drinkers consequently experience a diminution in the amount and quality of restfulness of their sleep.

Recovering alcoholics may experience months of insomnia as the brain overreacts to the absence of the depressant effect of alcohol. My friend, Bud, had a year of sleeplessness following his recovery.

In the most severe form, this reflex hyperactivity of the brain following withdrawal of alcohol produces a severe reaction called delirium tremens, commonly called "D.T.s" Within hours of removal of alcohol, the abstinent alcoholic begins to tremble and then to shake. This is the rebound hyperactivity of motor nerves, so long depressed by alcohol. In the most severe cases, the muscular hyperactivity will progress to grand mal seizures, or "rum fits." Untreated, they may be fatal.

The sensory nerves, no longer depressed, report all manner of unusual sensations: itching, burning, or aggravating feelings like ants crawling on the skin. The higher centers of the brain go haywire: abstinent alcoholics are confused, having no grasp on reality and no orientation in time and space. Visual and auditory hallucinations are common.

Alcoholics who have suffered serious withdrawal untreated never want to repeat the experience. The least bit of shaking necessitates a stiff drink to get the blood alcohol up quickly and bathe those neurons with the two-carbon depressant to which they are habituated.

It is a depressingly realistic way of life for many chronic alcoholics.

ALCOHOLIC ENCEPHALOPATHY

Reuben was back again. I could see the polished mahogany top of his bald pate on the gurney and the bright yellow of the fluid in his IV. They spiked his D5W (5 percent dextrose in water) with Berocca-C, a mix of B vitamins with vitamin C—a taxicab-yellow fluid clearly indicating to any passing medical staff that the patient was a severe chronic alcoholic. Reuben had such severe deficiencies that he had almost died twice.

Reuben suffered from Wernicke's encephalopathy. It is an intense disruption of brain function due to vitamin deficiencies caused by severe alcoholism. The B vitamins, in particular B_1 or thiamine, are critical enzymes in the metabolism of glucose. Unlike other parts of the body, which can metabolize fats and proteins, the brain and spinal cord can only burn glucose for fuel. That's why low blood sugar causes loss of consciousness and grand mal seizures. Alcoholics are deficient in B vitamins for three reasons. First, they ingest many of their calories from alcohol, neglecting their intake of vitamins. Second, they require more B vitamins than nonalcoholics because their daily intake of alcohol requires additional B vitamins to metabolize. Third, chronic alcoholism reduces the production and absorption of many vitamins from the intestine, including the B vitamins.

Wernicke's encephalopathy has a 20 percent fatality rate in emergency rooms. Brain and spinal cord cells, called neurons, are very unhappy when they don't have enough glucose. In mild to moderate deficiency states, they malfunction but the damage is reversible. In severe chronic cases, the neurons die and the injuries are permanent.

Reuben was a textbook example of the manifestations of severe chronic thiamine deficiency as they affect the central nervous system. Neuronal injury in the cerebrum or higher centers of the brain produced confusion, disorientation, and a severe loss of memory. I had admitted Reuben twice before and he had no recollection of me or what day or month it was. He also had been admitted twice in coma, but both times the Berocca-C had revived him.

Involvement of Reuben's cerebellum, the balance and coordination centers of the brain, produced a staggering broad-based gait (when he could walk) and inability to do simple things such as touching his nose with his fingertip. (I wondered how he could get a bottle to his mouth!) Reuben's cranial nerves were severely involved as is often the case. Damage to the muscles that control facial expression, eye movement, and vision caused partial paralysis of his eye muscles, particularly the abductors (those that look to the sides), so his eyes were continually crossed. Imbalance and weakness of his eye muscles also created a twitching movement of the eyeball called nystagmus. Temporary horizontal nystagmus is a sign of acute intoxication used by police officers when they do field sobriety tests. Reuben's nystagmus was horizontal and vertical, and it was permanent.

Reuben also had involvement of peripheral nerves causing a polyneuropathy: numbness, tingling, and burning. Interestingly, peripheral neuropathy, relatively common in seniors, is indistinguishable from alcohol-induced neuropathy. It is possible that many such cases result from heavy "social drinking."

Reuben recovered again with Berocca-C. But he died a month later on a similar admission of heart failure. The sympathetic nerves, which control the tiny muscles in the body's blood vessels, were damaged beyond repair. This caused the muscles to relax, creating a massive dilation of blood vessels. The heart can't pump fast enough to fill such a vastly increased vascular volume. Shock and death ensued.

The shiny brown pate and the lifesaving bottle of Berocca-C were gone. But the lessons he taught a whole decade of medical students and interns about alcohol deficiency states and the catastrophic effect on the brain were not lost on this student.

A description and discussion of the most devastating effects of alcohol on the brain and spinal cord might seem out of place in this book. But if alcohol is toxic to neurons and a lot of alcohol does a huge amount of damage, isn't it logical that low-level injury on a long-term basis would produce significant damage as well? Is the peripheral neuropathy seen increasingly in seniors due to heavy "social drinking"? Is the unsteadiness of old age in part due to cerebellar damage from alcohol? Is the cognitive impairment and memory loss so prevalent in seniors due, in part, to chronic alcohol toxicity?

The answers are probably yes. In a recent study of the elderly, more brain atrophy (shrinkage), as manifested by enlargement of fluid-filled spaces in the brain called ventricles, was seen in drinkers than in nondrinkers (Enzinger 2005)—incriminating evidence, relegated to the back pages of the daily news.

ALCOHOLIC HEPATITIS

Bart was quite upset when the blood bank refused to allow him to donate blood because of what they called his hepatitis. Bart is in his mid-fifties and has been a regular blood donor since his late twenties. His name appears on the five-gallon donor plaque and he aspired to have it on the ten-gallon plaque as well. No chance now as the blood bank will no longer accept him as a donor. His liver enzymes were elevated in last month's blood sample. Bart has since been to his personal physician and had a comprehensive panel of blood tests. He was negative for hepatitis A, B, and C, for mononucleosis, and for HIV, but the blood bank still refuses his blood. They can't risk giving a patient a unit of blood that may contain an infectious form of hepatitis as yet unknown. Having transmitted hundreds of thousands of cases of hepatitis C and HIV to unwitting blood recipients before adequate screening tests were developed, blood banks are now very cautious. There are other strains of HIV and hepatitis for which we have no adequate tests to date, so it's safer to exclude those individuals who have elevated liver enzymes from the donor pool. Bart will never make the ten-gallon club, but not because he has a new strain of hepatitis. His drinking has increased lately, resulting in elevated liver enzymes on the screening test for his last unit of donated blood.

Alcohol is a cell poison as is acetaldehyde, the first breakdown product in the metabolism of alcohol. Even in small doses, alcohol injures and kills liver cells. This causes them to leak the enzymes that enable them to process digested material such as proteins, fats, and carbohydrates and to detoxify harmful substances that have been ingested. Liver enzymes can be measured in a blood sample. When they are elevated from the normally low levels, it means that the liver is suffering some ongoing damage. The general term for any inflammation of the liver is "hepatitis." The term does not imply an infectious origin, although people interpret it that way. It actually denotes any process that results in injury to liver cells with the attendant inflammation. The various forms of hepatitis that are caused by microorganisms are labeled "infectious hepatitis."

Every time Bart has a glass of wine, he has a small episode of hepatitis. Liver cells are injured and some die, releasing their enzymes. The liver is a remarkably resilient organ. As much as 90 percent of the liver can be surgically removed and the remainder will, in part, regenerate. But with alcohol and other substances that are toxic to the liver, it is not analogous to removing a hunk of liver and leaving a healthy piece to regenerate. Rather, alcohol causes diffuse injury and death to liver cells, resulting in the formation of scar tissue, or "fibrosis." Fibrosis changes the very complex and intricate way in which the liver functions. The liver cells, the bile ducts, and the portal veins are all arranged in a precise manner so that the liver can do its job of metabolizing nutrients and detoxifying harmful substances both formed within the body (such as ammonia) and introduced extrinsically (such as drugs, environmental toxins, or alcohol). The fibrosis that results from alcohol injury to liver cells alters this intricate architecture so that different component cells don't hook up properly to do their job. The short-term result is a liver that is compromised in its ability to perform its jobs. The long-term result is a liver that develops the extreme form of fibrosis known as "cirrhosis," rendering it incapable of functioning efficiently and resulting in liver failure with its myriad medical complications.

Drinking is such a socially acceptable and culturally ingrained activity that most people ignore its contribution to serious liver damage. Patients who are wary of taking certain medications because they have a "risk" of causing liver damage always amuse me. There is a very effective oral medication for athlete's foot and toenail fungus, for instance, that has a chance of producing liver toxicity in one-tenth of 1 percent of the people who take it. The hepatitis is mild to moderate and completely reversible when the drug is stopped. And yet, when I present to patients the option of taking this drug, at least half will say, "Oh, no, doctor. I don't want to take anything that has a risk of damaging my liver." Many of these same patients had two highballs before dinner and split a bottle of wine with their spouse the night before, not aware that the damage caused by alcohol has the same potential seriousness as that caused by medication. Some more addicted patients are unwilling or unable to restrict their alcohol intake while taking antifungal medication.

Do other medications cause hepatitis? Yes. Medications with potential liver toxicity include those prescribed for high blood pressure, high cholesterol, seizure disorders, cardiac arrhythmias, and arthritis. Blood thinners, antibiotics, and other prescription drugs can also affect liver function. Conscientious physicians almost always discuss potential side effects with their patients before they prescribe medications. The patient listens attentively and reassures the doctor that she only has "a glass of wine with dinner" and will abstain, which she does, for a while. But when she has a couple of glasses of champagne at a wedding with no reaction, she adds a glass of wine with dinner, and five years after the medication was prescribed, she has forgotten the admonition about drinking. She is ingesting two hepatotoxic (liver-toxic) substances; if she is taking additional medication, she may be ingesting even more.

Alcoholism is epidemic in our senior population. A significant number of seniors are bored or depressed, oftentimes they have suffered a loss and are grieving, and many are in chronic pain from arthritis or back problems. As a result, seniors tend to drink, or to drink more, although alcohol enhances depression instead of improving it and is a lousy pain medication.

In due time, seniors no longer drink for pain relief, for depression, or for a pick-me-up. Now they drink because they have to, because they cannot stop. Unwittingly, they have learned the truth about alcohol.

It is powerfully addictive.

ALCOHOL, OBESITY, AND DIABETES

The love handles and beer belly were impressive. Harry was in for a long-overdue checkup, and his mid-fifties frame was woefully overburdened. Five feet eleven and 220 pounds, Harry's list of medical problems read like a litany of risk factors for an early demise: hypertension, coronary artery disease, diabetes, and elevated triglycerides. In actuality, he had only one problem. He drank too much.

The body treats alcohol as if it were a sugar, or a simple carbohydrate. Beer, often referred to as a "liquid sandwich," tallies 150 calories of pure carbohydrates. When you drink a six-pack of beer, it's similar to eating 900 calories of sugar. But instead of a sugar high, you get intoxicated.

Carbohydrates are the high-octane fuel of the body, used by the muscles for strenuous exercise. Glucose, which is the simplest of the carbohydrates, is the sole usable source of energy for the brain. The body has a limited ability to store carbohydrates. It packs away a little in muscles for a burst of energy in emergencies, and it stores some in the liver. In both venues, carbohydrate is stored in a long chain of glucose molecules linked together called glycogen. Any excess carbohydrate the body is unable to burn for its daily energy requirement *is converted into fat!* Long chains of carbohydrates are converted into fat and attached to a three-carbon molecule called glycerin, producing one of the dangerous fats in the bloodstream, triglycerides. The result of eating too much sugar, or drinking too much alcohol, is elevated triglyceride levels in the blood.

Triglycerides, originating from excess sugar intake, contribute heavily to arteriosclerosis, as does cholesterol, which originates from animal fat.

Let's get back to Harry. The spare tire around his middle is referred to as a "glucose-meter" by physicians specializing in diabetes. Fat accumulating there is predominantly caused by excess sugar (alcohol, carbohydrate) in the diet. Since insulin can be diluted by fat, there may not be enough to maintain a normal blood sugar. The result is obesity-onset or type 2 diabetes.

Harry's nightly six-pack represents 900 calories of carbohydrate. A pound of fat represents roughly 3,000 calories, so Harry's six-pack creates almost a third-pound of fat.

America's love affair with alcohol is one factor in the obesity epidemic in our culture. It also accounts for a frightening increase in heart disease and hypertension from the elevated triglycerides, and type 2 diabetes.

When I quit drinking, I lost eight pounds and one inch off my waistline within several months. I also stopped having very troubling bouts of hypoglycemia, or low blood sugar. I used to get shaky and weak an hour or so after eating a doughnut, cookie, or anything with concentrated sugar. The intake of sugar produces an overly brisk release of insulin, which rapidly drops the blood sugar, producing the wobbliness. When the liver is functioning properly, it stores glycogen, which serves as an emergency supply of glucose to prevent attacks of hypoglycemia. When the blood sugar drops from the insulin release, the liver breaks down glycogen into glucose units and releases it into the bloodstream to mitigate the impending hypoglycemia. Alcohol prevents the liver from storing glycogen. Unwittingly, I had been causing my hypoglycemia by drinking.

ALCOHOL AND THE HEART

George was blowing bubbles. Not Double Bubble or Bazooka and not the soapy stuff in the bottle. His bubbles were small and tinged with blood.

George arrived at my medical admitting ward as a "red blanket," a red sheet covering the gurney to denote his critical condition. He was desperately short of breath; his respiration was like the chug of a steam locomotive. Extremely agitated, he grabbed at my sleeve, pulling me toward him. He was experiencing one of the classical symptoms of advanced heart failure, the "feeling of impending doom."

I went right to work. An oxygen mask was immediately fitted over his face, and rotating tourniquets were placed on his extremities to sequester some of the excess fluid to take the load off his heart. He was given morphine, furosemide (a powerful diuretic), and ouabain (a fast-acting digitalis), all intravenously.

Within ten minutes, the medications were working. George was calmer. His respiratory and pulse rates were slowing. He had urinated over a liter. And, he was no longer blowing bubbles.

We saved him again. But he would be back, as his heart was in terrible condition. He had alcoholic cardiomyopathy, a disease of the heart muscle caused by alcohol.

We are told that alcohol is good for the heart, that it makes the heart healthier. But we are only told what they want us to know. It's a dosage thing. In small quantities, alcohol may be good for the heart, although, particularly with wine, it may not be the alcohol but another ingredient that is beneficial. In higher dosages, alcohol is toxic to the myocardium or heart muscle. Over time, it may produce a severe weakening of the muscle that can result in a scenario that George and thousands of alcoholics like him experience up to five times before succumbing to congestive heart failure.

We are unaware of alcoholic cardiomyopathy because the alcohol lobby controls very carefully what appears in the national media about alcohol. What does appear often has a positive slant: alcohol lowers your blood pressure, improves your memory, decreases your cholesterol, and is good for your heart.

The sound and print bites regarding alcohol in national media coverage are very carefully orchestrated. Papers from the prestigious *New England Journal of Medicine* or the *Journal of the American Medical Association* are quoted, giving scientific credence to the claims of the benefits of drinking alcohol. All that appears is a two-line conclusion of a very complex study funded by a grant from some wine institute that may be flawed in its design. The headline states "Drinking Improves Heart Disease Survival." Excluded is that the study's definition of drinking is one glass of red wine (one and a half ounces of alcohol) a day, three times a week. High-functioning alcoholics who drank a liter of wine with dinner last night feel confident and smug that drinking is good for their health.

Not so.

You need to hear the rest of the story.

The studies that I note in this section on the health risks of alcohol are referenced at the end of the book by author. These citations represent just a small portion of the literature on the adverse health effects of drinking alcohol. None of them made headline news. None of them were funded by the liquor industry.

Let's get back to alcohol and heart disease. What are the facts? The landmark study cited as proof that alcohol promotes heart health is a study that compares the French with Americans. The study showed that France has a lower incidence of heart disease, although their diet is higher in fat, a contradiction christened "the French Paradox." A closer look revealed that the French had a much higher consumption of wine than did the Americans. The initial conclusion was that consumption of alcohol, particularly in the form of red wine, was protective against the development of heart disease. Further study showed that a peculiar compound in the skin of grapes known as resveratrol may be the beneficial substance.

But there's more to the story that was never published. Let's call it "the French Conundrum." Although the French die less of heart disease, they succumb more frequently to cancer and suicide than Americans. The cancer is promoted by the acetaldehyde formed from the alcohol, and interestingly enough, resveratrol may also be responsible. It has estrogen-like properties and may be, in part, the cause of the increase in breast cancer in red-wine-drinking women

The increase in suicide may be the result of the aggravation of severe depression caused by alcohol.

This information never reached the American public. With selective filtration of the facts, the liquor industry continues to advocate alcohol as a beneficial part of a healthful diet. Moderate and heavy drinkers, with denial and rationalization fully operational, proclaim alcohol to be the fountain of youth.

In stark contrast, the American public is outraged by the health hazards caused by tobacco use. Class action suits, public service announcements, prohibition of smoking in public places, and health warnings on packages attest to the increased public awareness and sentiment against tobacco use. Like alcohol lobbyists today, tobacco lobbyists at one time hid the devastating health risks from the public.

Alcohol is contributory to eight different types of cancer and to gastroesophageal reflux disease. Its role in producing fetal alcohol syndrome accounts for 20 percent of the money spent for the treatment of mental retardation in this country; it is a leading cause of osteoporosis, suppresses the immune system, and is a major factor in highway deaths, spousal and child abuse, and homicide.

Smokers harm only themselves and their immediate family through second-hand exposure. Alcohol harms randomly on the streets and highways of America and, in an ever-widening circle, the family and friends of the alcoholic.

So why doesn't the package labeling on alcoholic beverages really reflect the extent of these hazards?

It does, sort of:

"**Government Warning:** *(1) According to the surgeon general, women should not drink alcoholic beverages during pregnancy because of the risk of birth defects. (2) Consumption of alcoholic beverages impairs your ability to drive a car or operate machinery, and may cause health problems.*"

Why isn't the public better informed? Why isn't the warning more explicit? Because of the power and money of the alcohol industry.

WES

My friend Wes told me that, at his worst, he filled a tumbler with vodka, put a straw in it, and set it on his nightstand when he staggered into bed at night. That way he could get his blood alcohol back up quickly in the morning to avoid withdrawal.

8

DYING FROM CHRONIC ALCOHOL POISONING

Bruce Anderson was gazing at death as he stared up at me with terror in his eyes. His lids were drawn back and the globes almost bulged out of their sockets. His sclerae were the color of a crook-necked squash, jaundiced from the bilirubin in his bloodstream that a failing liver could not metabolize and remove.

Bruce was in hard restraints—heavy leather hand and ankle cuffs strapped to the frame of the bed so he couldn't flail about or pull out the tubes and IVs that were keeping him alive. A football helmet was strapped on, with a large rubber tube that entered his nose and went down into his stomach tied to the nose guard. He shook violently from D.T.s, from the chill of the ice water that was being flushed down the tube, and from shock, having lost a third of his blood volume to GI (gastrointestinal) bleeding.

Anderson was an alcoholic in the end stages of liver failure and was bleeding from esophageal varices. It was his first bleed. There was a fifty-fifty chance it would be his last. His beard was caked with clotted blood, his hair was matted, and his arms were covered with large purple bruises.

How did this happen to him?

One word.

Alcohol.

Bruce was thirty-nine years old. He began drinking in college, with the seemingly harmless drinking games and bacchanalian rites of fraternity life. He graduated in engineering and then took a job as a technical sales rep for a medical device company. His work included dining potential customers. The two-scotch-and-water lunches and dinners on the company expense account were gradually preceded by a couple of beers in the bar and followed by a snifter of brandy and a cigar after dessert. Bruce made a lot of sales. He was a good talker, even while drunk, and clients liked his humor and friendly manner. He was a high-function-ing alcoholic.

Bruce met and married a flight attendant, Jeannie. They were perfect together: she drank gin and tonics and became very sexy when she drank. They had an elegant townhouse in Marina del Rey and a small sailboat. Life was rosy, but short-lived.

It lasted eighteen months. Jeannie was late returning from a three-day trip. Two weeks late. When she returned, it was to tell Bruce that she had fallen in love (over gin and tonics) with a pilot named Carl, and she was leaving. Bruce went on a bender. He missed work for a week, and when he came back, the humor and friendliness had been replaced by irony and sarcasm. The two-scotch-and-water lunches became three-martini lunches, and if he did return to work after lunch, he just shuffled papers on his desk. His sales fell off. Clients were put off by his bitter sarcasm and grew tired of hearing how Jeannie had ruined his life. After three months in a self-destructive decline, Bruce was fired. He went on another bender and ended up in the county hospital detox unit. He was assigned a social worker, given a referral to a rehabilitation program, and sent home.

Bruce lost his townhouse and moved in with his brother. On his budget he could no longer afford scotch, so he drank cheap vodka. He found a job as a janitor in an office building downtown, but after repeated absences, they let him go. His brother finally threw him out and he went to live with his widowed diabetic mother. When she died, he found himself on the street. Bruce had made the transition from a high-functioning alcoholic to a common drunk.

It took eleven years for the alcohol to ruin his liver. Little by little, high concentrations of alcohol killed liver cells. They were replaced by fibrous tissue. Gradually, the beautifully complex liver was turned into a rock-hard mass of scar tissue, and Bruce developed cirrhosis.

Understanding the process that produces liver cirrhosis and all of the many medical problems that result requires knowledge of basic liver structure and function. The liver, ("hepar" in Latin) is a large (three-pound) organ that sits under the right diaphragm. Its jobs are legion: it receives all the incoming nutrients from the gut through a special set of veins called the portal system. Digested food is absorbed through the intestinal wall into small veins that travel to the liver. Here, the nutrients are metabolized by liver cells into usable proteins, fats, and carbohydrates. These then enter the general circulation, to be used by the body. The liver also detoxifies any hazardous substances or drugs that may be absorbed from the intestine. It is like a huge manufacturing and recycling center. It recycles the vital blood-carrying protein hemoglobin by accepting a by-product called bilirubin and altering it to produce the substance bile, which flows through ducts to the gall bladder where it is excreted back into the gut periodically to help digest fats. Finally, a network of immune cells in the liver are responsible for gobbling up foreign proteins, bacteria, and parasites in the blood that might be attacking the body.

When alcohol is absorbed through the gut wall, it travels to the liver where it damages liver cells (hepatocytes), producing varying degrees of inflammation termed alcoholic hepatitis. Hepatocytes are actually killed, and in the resultant cleanup effort, they may regenerate but the complicated connections to the incoming portal veins, bile ducts, and nutrient arteries are often disrupted. If severe enough, fibrosis or scarring occurs, and the complex architecture of this miraculous organ may be altered. With repeated episodes of alcoholic hepatitis, the scarring gradually narrows the incoming or portal veins. At some point, when the scarring is severe, the liver cannot adequately process the incoming portal blood from the intestine and the blood backs up, the scarred liver producing a tourniquet effect on the portal veins. The resultant increased pressure in these veins causes them to bulge, and when stretched to the extreme, they may rupture. The internal varicose veins or varices thus created line the gut, including the esophagus, stomach, bowel, and rectum. Internal hemorrhoidal as well as esophageal varicose veins are the result of this high pressure in the portal system, a condition known as portal hypertension.

The massively dilated veins that line the esophagus are the most prone to bleed. Sharp-edged foods like potato chips or a fishbone might scratch the mucosal lining over one of these varices or they might tear from the violent vomiting of acute alcohol intoxication. The instant these veins rupture, at least a quart of blood under pressure fills the stomach. Some is digested into a black, tarry ooze called melena that smells like death itself. Most is vomited as bright red blood.

Varices are thin-walled and, unlike arteries, have little or no muscle in their walls. As a result, when shock sets in, there is no compensatory spasm of the muscular wall of the varices to stop the bleeding. They just bleed until there is no more blood in them. Not uncommonly, "GI bleeders" that are due to cirrhosis and varices "bleed out," or exsanguinate. Fatal shock and cardiac arrest quickly follow.

Bruce Anderson was bleeding out. When he arrived in my emergency medicine admitting ward as a red blanket, his pulse was rapid and thready, his blood pressure almost nonexistent. He had a large gauge tube cut down into the vein in his forearm that had been placed in the emergency room before he was shipped upstairs, and he had already been given two liters of Ringer's lactate and two units of untyped, uncrossed whole blood. There was no time to type the blood. He would have died without it.

My job was to pass the Sengstaken-Blakemore tube. It was huge, but with KY jelly in Bruce's nostril and some luck, I got it down. It had a doughnutlike balloon just in front of the stomach end, and it could be inflated by a small tube that ran along the sidewall of the larger tube. I quickly filled the balloon with mercury, used for its weight. Once the balloon was inflated, I drew back on the tube, trying to make a seal around the cardio-esophageal junction, the neck of the esophagus as it enters the stomach. This is where esophageal varices most commonly bleed. Hopefully, this would press on, or tamponade, and stop the bleeding.

It stopped for a while and we were able to stabilize Bruce's blood pressure. With the acute emergency over, I was able to complete my physical exam.

Bruce was a textbook on the physical findings of end-stage liver disease due to alcoholism. He was jaundiced from the failing liver. The bilirubin could not be conjugated or processed by the failing liver, so it backed up in the blood and stained all the tissues of the body including his skin and eyeballs. Because his liver could not manufacture bile to digest the fat in his diet, his stool was a whitish clay color. His skin was covered with large red bumps called spider hemangiomas, which are small arteries that grew into the skin as a result of an excessive amount of estrogen in Bruce's blood. Estrogen is normally produced by the adrenal gland and broken down by the liver. Without a functioning liver, Bruce's body had excess estrogen, which was also responsible for Bruce's large breasts and shrunken, almost absent testicles. So much for the myth that alcohol increases your libido. Bruce hadn't had an erection in five years.

He shivered from the shock of blood loss and the ice water lavaging his stomach. There was a coarser shake also, perhaps the first sign of impending delirium tremens. And there was yet a third movement, a slower, rhythmic cadence as his feet and hands patted the mattress. This "liver flap" was produced by large amounts of ammonia in Bruce's blood. A normal by-product of metabolism, especially of proteins, ammonia is usually broken down and detoxified by the liver. Bruce's liver was no longer able to detoxify anything.

Bruce had a protuberant belly, caused in part by his enlarged, rock-hard liver and by a massive accumulation of fluid in the abdominal cavity. The same congestion and back pressure that created the portal hypertension also caused the liver to weep fluid, known as ascites, and his belly was full of it.

I finished my exam and was charting my findings when the bottom dropped out. Bruce's blood pressure plummeted and, sensing impending doom, he began to thrash and writhe uncontrollably.

A death struggle can be a terrifying event to witness for the first time. Our inner primitive animal fights, often with superhuman strength and violence, to survive. So it was with Bruce. I watched, riveted, as every muscle fought against the restraints, bowing the steel rails of the bed to which they were anchored. Struggling to sit up as far as his bonds would allow, he growled a guttural sound, an utterance of anguish and fear. His fingers grasped for anything and clung with a death grip to the sheets and railing. His eyes, tightly shut with effort, suddenly opened and looked directly into mine. The look was of desperation and fear. Death hovered at the foot of his bed, and he was powerless to drive it away. Then the connection was lost, his eyes closed again, and he was abandoned to the mindless animalistic struggle. I turned the IV line wide open and hung another unit of uncrossed blood. The return from the nasogastric tube was pure blood. I tightened the tension on the tube, but as I did, his pulse disappeared, his bulging yellow eyes rolled back in his head, the thrashing ceased, and his yellow skin turned blue.

An hour later, after CPR, fluids, blood, and intracardiac epinephrine, Bruce Anderson got his wish. He had finally killed himself.

In the intern's sleeping room, I looked at myself in the mirror. There was exhaustion in my eyes. My face was spattered with dried blood. There were bloody fingerprints on my shirt where Bruce had tried, in his final agony, to get my attention, to somehow convey to me the terror he was feeling. To swear that now, finally, he could quit.

Jim Wells

I received an e-mail from an old college buddy last night. He reported that Jim Wells died last week of alcoholic liver failure. A brilliant athlete, an all-American volleyball player, Jim was one of the best setters in the game. He was a year ahead of me in school. A little blond-haired surfer dude, he had grown up playing beach volleyball in Manhattan Beach.

No telling when he started drinking.

I thought of all the end-stage alcoholics I have seen, all the terminal cirrhotics. I couldn't imagine Jim, that fresh-faced kid, with a huge protruding belly from the ascites, red blotchy spiders over his face and trunk. I wondered how he died. Did he bleed out from esophageal varices or just slip into hepatic coma and die of pneumonia? What did he think when he realized he was dying? Looking back, he was drunk a lot in college, at almost every party and all the weekend nights. But so was everybody else. Jim didn't stand out as the worst drinker in the fraternity. But obviously the pattern that he established in high school and college continued unabated or worsened throughout his adult life.

And it killed him.

9

DYING OF ACUTE ALCOHOL POISONING

One minute he was alive, talking about a mountain bike trip and plans for the holidays. Ninety minutes later he was dead. Two fine young men killed themselves with alcohol in our town last year. One lived out by the state park where we ride our horses, and every time we trailer out there, I read a banner stretched on a fence along the road.

WE MISS YOU, RANDY!

And I mourn.

Randy was a junior in high school. He and his buddy cut school and went to a friend's house to do some serious drinking. Incredibly, the friend's parents were home part of the time and knew or should have known what was going on.

They had stolen a half-gallon of whiskey from one of their parents' liquor cabinet. They began to drink.

The drink of choice for killing oneself with alcohol is hard liquor simply because it has a much higher concentration of alcohol than beer or wine. The alcohol builds up in the bloodstream faster, causing deadly poisoning before the side effects prevent or reduce the intake. It is possible to kill yourself with beer, but the lower concentration (6 percent or 12 proof [1 percent = 2 proof]) requires the consumption of much larger quantities. Before a fatal blood alcohol is reached, the beer drinker may mercifully vomit or pass out. The same is true of wine, which, at 10 to 12 percent alcohol (20 to 24 proof), requires the drinker to consume a larger quantity than hard liquor. With 80 proof whiskey, 100 proof vodka or tequila, 151 proof rum, or 198 proof grain alcohol ("white lightning" or "Everclear"), it is a much shorter journey into oblivion.

So when you are matching your friend drink for drink, guzzling several ounces of straight whiskey each time, you need to remember one critical fact. You can drink and absorb alcohol much faster than your liver and other tissues can metabolize and get rid of it, so the level is constantly rising. If it reaches 0.4 percent before you pass out, vomit, or somebody stops you, you may just die. Randy did.

There is a dynamic process going on when you consume alcohol. There is consumption, absorption, and elimination. Alcohol is absorbed rather quickly and at almost 100 percent efficiency, so consumption is roughly equal to absorption. Elimination is variable but within a relatively narrow range. The novice drinker can metabolize one to one and a half ounces of alcohol per hour. A veteran drinker, whose liver has had repeated exposures to alcohol and is more efficient, may be able to metabolize half again that much; however, there is a limit to how fast alcohol can be cleared from the body. That upper limit may approach two ounces per hour. The blood alcohol level (BAL) depends on how fast the alcohol is consumed and how strong it is.

When large amounts of highly concentrated alcohol are consumed quickly, the normal stages of drunkenness are passed through, but very rapidly because the drug is being consumed and absorbed at such a high rate. And as a high school junior, you're not an everyday drinker, so your liver is not habituated; it doesn't metabolize the alcohol efficiently. Your friend is the same height but weighs fifteen pounds more, mostly fat. Because alcohol is evenly distributed in tissues, he can drink 15 percent more than you can for each stage of intoxication.

At 0.1 percent blood alcohol (allowing for elimination of an ounce and a half an hour, that is an accumulation of four ounces of alcohol, eight ounces of whiskey), you are pleasantly buzzed. You feel lighthearted and happy. You're talkative and funny. All your worries seem trivial and you have a warm glow. Your lips might feel a little thick and your balance might not be perfect, but you could probably pass a field sobriety test. You would fail a blood or urine alcohol test and a Breathalyzer because the legal limit for alcohol is 0.08 percent. You are feeling good.

At 0.2 percent blood alcohol (a net surplus of eight ounces of alcohol, sixteen ounces of whiskey) as a rookie, you are feeling very drunk. Your speech is slurred and your walk is quite unsteady. You may see double. You are not as mellow as you were and become loud and obnoxious, as normal social restraint is dissolved by the liquor. Males may still be able to get an erection but it probably won't be a great one. And there might be real difficulty having an orgasm. You're just plain drunk.

Veteran drinkers may function surprisingly well at 0.2 percent. Their livers have increased enzymes for breaking down the alcohol, and both nerves and muscles have learned to adapt to higher levels of ethanol while still functioning adequately. Many high-functioning alcoholics live their entire waking lives with a blood alcohol of 0.2 percent. They drive, work, close big business deals, get pregnant, have kids, and, in time, can't function without it.

A friend of my parents, Jack McDougall, became enormously successful drinking a fifth of bourbon every working day, and more on weekends. The boardrooms of the Fortune 500 companies are well stocked with high-functioning alcoholics who can and do function remarkably well with blood alcohols of nearly 0.2 percent. It's a given that they will have two drinks during a power lunch with prospective clients, pour a drink from their sideboard in the afternoon when they clinch the deal, stop at a bar across the street from the office before they leave for home, and have a couple of double highballs before dinner. It would stagger the imagination to know what proportion of high-level business executives are also high-functioning alcoholics.

After twelve ounces of alcohol (a net gain of twenty-four ounces of whiskey), the blood alcohol climbs to 0.3 percent and the staggering drunk falls down. Alcohol affects the higher centers of the brain first, that is, the cerebral thinking, reasoning, remembering, and emoting part of the brain. At increased blood levels, the mid-portion of the brain, the cerebellum, is affected, impairing balance and coordination. At yet higher levels of alcohol, the lower centers of the brain are affected as well. These are in the brain stem, which is in charge of consciousness, blood pressure, respiration, and temperature regulation. When the blood alcohol reaches 0.3 percent, most people pass out. If they are lucky enough to be in a temperate environment, a knowledgeable and caring soul may turn their head to the side to prevent them from choking on or aspirating their vomit. If they are unlucky and pass out alone in the cold, they could suffer hypothermia or freeze to death, as alcohol impairs temperature control and dilates capillaries close to the surface of the skin. They quickly lose their core heat to the surrounding cold and suffer hypothermia. Although my emergency room work occurred in a temperate climate zone, it was common to see drunks brought in comatose with body temperatures in the low nineties.

Unconscious, the drunk may vomit, plugging his airway, or worse, the vomit may be aspirated or sucked into his lungs. The effect of stomach acid and food particles is devastating on lung tissue, causing aspiration pneumonia. If not fatal, it may cause severe scarring and permanent reduction of functional lung tissue.

In a coma, the drunk may be insensitive to the damaging effect of hard surfaces on soft tissues resting upon them. A conscious or sleeping person shifts position when pressure on an area of skin becomes uncomfortable. A passed-out drunk does not. The result is pressure sores on the skin and occasional massive areas of necrosis or dead muscle and subcutaneous tissue.

After a net surplus of sixteen ounces of alcohol (thirty-two ounces of whiskey), a blood alcohol of 0.4 percent is reached, and death may follow. I say "may" because with some veteran alcoholics, it may take a bit more. I was an intern at LA County-USC Medical Center during a severe flu epidemic. A reorganization of medical admitting had created an overdose ward, exclusively for "doses" to take the pressure off the overcrowding of the hospital with flu cases. Along with another intern, I was selected to staff the "dose" ward. One night, I admitted a comatose drunk, named Billy, who was well-known to the staff. I worked him up, started an IV, and drew some blood. He was stable and quiet in the corner of the admitting room when my attention turned to a new patient, a famous actor who had some heroin at a party that was much more potent than he anticipated. He was comatose and in respiratory arrest. By the time I had stabilized our celebrity, I looked over to see that Billy was gone. He had disconnected his IV and left without saying good-bye. Then the lab called with his blood alcohol. It was 0.45 percent. We all just shook our heads. Billy set the record for blood alcohol during my tenure on the overdose ward. Just then the phone rang from the ER. They were sending up a "red blanket." The elevator doors opened, and under the red sheet was a moribund Billy. Apparently, he passed out again on the front steps of the hospital. When security found him, he was not breathing. A little CPR, an endotracheal tube, an ambu bag, and another IV, and Billy was mine again. I was able to bring him back, but alcohol finally killed him several months later on another intern's watch.

Randy and his friend shared a half-gallon of whiskey. That's sixty-four ounces of liquor, thirty-two ounces of alcohol, and it killed him. He drank it so fast that he was able to reach 0.4 percent before he passed out, he got sick, or someone stopped him. When he finally did pass out, the alcohol level was so high that it stopped his breathing. Without oxygen, a heart already weakened by high alcohol levels cannot last long, perhaps a minute or two. Then it stops. And tragically, no one recognized what had happened in time to help. So, the world lost another young person to alcohol. Another bright and promising future that would not be. Another devastated family. Another memorial service warning friends about binge drinking. Another obituary chronicling the life of a "nice guy…promising student...gifted athlete." And another sign on a fence—a memorial to a moment of bad judgment.

10

LESSER-KNOWN HEALTH PROBLEMS DUE TO ALCOHOL

George was back in the hospital again. His temperature was 102.5° F. His eyes watered down his pink, puffy face. Beefy red patches covered his forehead and scalp and nearly 50 percent of the rest of his body. The remainder was pink and swollen almost to the point of weeping: generalized, erythrodermic psoriasis. He was toxic, and he was drunk.

Physicians have observed over many years that almost every rash is worse if the patient is a heavy drinker. When I worked at the VA hospital during my residency, and subsequently, when I was teaching, I continually observed the high correlation between people with bad psoriasis or eczema and heavy drinking. Long philosophical discussions resulted, as we debated the question of whether alcoholics with the genetic predisposition develop psoriasis or whether the stigma of bad psoriasis makes people drunks.

It may be difficult to understand this question if you have never seen severe psoriasis. It causes large raised pink-to-red scaling patches of skin anywhere on the body. The elbows and knees are generally the worst, but the entire front of the leg and arm can be affected. The scalp is commonly involved, and the process resembles an industrial-strength case of dandruff or cradle cap. Uninitiated observers may be frightened by the appearance of a person with severe psoriasis. You wouldn't want him sitting next to you on the bus or in the dermatologist's waiting room.

People with psoriasis are very self-conscious about their appearance. Psychological studies have shown that they have a very poor self-image, an altered perception of their body. They are also more likely to have depression.

Interestingly, recent scientific studies have shown that psoriasis is caused by an alteration in the immune system. A subset of T lymphocytes are abnormal, the

Th1 lymphocytes. This leads to the abnormal production of messenger chemicals that increase inflammation, producing the pink scaly skin that we recognize as psoriasis.

Eczema, or atopic dermatitis, is a very itchy, scaly skin disease that has an allergic basis. It is commonly associated with hay fever, asthma, food allergies, and a history of other family members who have the same. It is even more common than psoriasis and, in its severe form, just as physically and socially debilitating. It turns out that eczema is caused by an alteration in another subset of T lymphocytes, the Th 2 lymphocytes. They produce a completely different group of messenger chemicals including an antibody called IgE, which is responsible for the release of histamine, the culprit chemical that produces the agonizing itch that is the hallmark of eczema.

Have you ever had a horrible itch? Poison oak? Scabies? People with eczema live with that kind of itch all the time.

So, why the lesson in dermatology?

Alcohol has been proven to enhance the alteration in both the Th-1 and Th-2 systems and acts as an amplifier of inflammation. It aggravates both psoriasis and eczema. And, as these conditions worsen, the psychological stress increases, the drinking increases, and the condition flares to a greater degree, creating a cycle of increasing intensity.

The abnormal antibody IgE, which causes the allergic symptoms in all three of the allergic triad (eczema, asthma, and hay fever), is greatly increased by intake of alcohol. A bad asthmatic needs to give up his nightly half-liter of wine.

It has long been observed that alcoholics get more infections and more unusual infections than the general population. It was thought that was due to the neglect of personal hygiene, inattention to minor problems before they become major, and the abnormal life circumstances produced by severe chronic alcoholism. But it's more than that. I see chronic intractable infections in successful businessmen who drink a lot. I see fungus infections that are resistant to treatment, and they seem anecdotally to be much more common in alcoholics than in nondrinkers.

This occurs because heavy drinkers are immune-suppressed. Their immune systems are not as robust as they would be in an alcohol-free environment.

The hard-drinking, successful businessman will not accept that the itchy pimples on his scalp are due to his heavy drinking. Most people are in denial about their drinking and they flat-out lie to me about their daily consumption. But, they want me to fix them. They don't want to modify any behaviors, especially giving up their two-martini lunches and the bottle of wine with dinner. They just want me to make them better. It is an interesting phenomenon. These are people who are used to being in control and getting what they want. They hold me personally responsible for their disease, and it's my responsibility to cure them. There must be a pill they can take, a salve they can apply. Sadly, it is a theme of much of our society's health woes. We don't want to change our diet or lifestyle; we just want a pill to fix it so we can keep on with the way we want to live. Patients with this mind-set are very hard to treat.

So, if alcohol decreases or alters immune function, and immune function is responsible for tumor surveillance, does that mean alcoholics more commonly get cancer?

Probably. That study has not been done, but it should be. Certainly, alcoholics get some cancers more commonly. As we discussed in chapter 8, mouth, throat, and esophageal cancers are much more common in people with heavy alcohol intake. Smoking and alcohol seem to be cofactors in all three of those diseases, but alcohol alone may serve to promote them in a number of people. Liver, colon, and breast cancers are known to be increased in people who drink alcohol. There is an increased probability that pancreatic cancer is also caused by alcohol intake, though the hard data is, as yet, unavailable. But in addition to the cancers known to be caused by alcohol, a generalized predisposition to all kinds of cancer may be brought about by the decrease in the vitality of the immune system due to chronic alcohol intake. And, as stated earlier, once cancer is present in the body, regular alcohol intake may promote its spread.

For the middle-aged woman, alcohol may aggravate many of the symptoms of menopause, especially the generalized dilation of blood vessels known as "hot flashes." The mechanism is simply the additive effect of dilation of blood vessels brought on by alcohol.

Considering the many negative health effects of alcohol, I am amazed that anyone would drink. Of course, many drinkers are unaware of the facts because they have not been well publicized. Hopefully this book will serve that end and will help to counter the barrage of alcohol lobby-generated press releases concerning the beneficial effects of alcohol. Then, well informed, people can choose to drink or not based on a full understanding of alcohol's benefits and risks.

11

UNSUSPECTED PREGNANCY BEGETS TRAGEDY: FETAL ALCOHOL SYNDROME

"Push down, Stacey."

Bearing down, she screamed in pain. The contraction lasted about thirty seconds.

"Now relax and breathe."

In labor for twelve hours and hard labor for the last two, Stacey was exhausted. But she was young and strong, and she desperately wanted this child.

Stacey and Tom were ecstatic about the prospect of their firstborn. They had been married five years, were established financially, had traveled, and, as Stacey put it, "had done the self-indulgent, selfish things" so that neither would resent the financial demand and time restraints of a new baby. Stacey took a leave of absence from her work as human resources director for the local community college. Tom's insurance business was thriving and could offset Stacey's loss of income.

Stacey rested from the intensity of the contraction. Despite the cramping pain, she could hardly contain her excitement. Both she and Tom had large families, and the cumulative anticipation of the blessed event, which had produced three baby showers and a phone network of relatives waiting to hear the news, was palpable.

Another contraction increased in intensity. Stacey gripped the rails of the table, her contorted face revealing the effort.

"There's a head, Stacey. Keep pushing."

"Oh, God." Stacey cried with the effort and some pain.

"Keep it up. That's it. Here he comes. Keep it coming." Dr. Johnson's skilled hands gently turned the head, sweeping the mouth and throat with a finger to clear it of debris, and delivered the shoulders, the torso, and finally the tiny hands and feet. He double-clamped the umbilical cord and separated it between the clamps, so focused on the task that he hadn't noticed the child as yet. He held the infant by the legs, spanked him on the buttocks to produce a hoarse cry, and then he placed the baby on Stacey's belly.

He was about to say, "Here's your healthy baby boy" when he noticed the face. He said nothing. The silence was deafening.

"What's wrong, Doctor?" Stacey knew something was wrong. Terror welled up within her.

Dr. Johnson silently stared. The facial features were unmistakable. The tiny face was flattened centrally, looking as if it had been pressed against a plate glass window. The cheeks had almost no curve to them and the upper lip was thin, without the delicate upward curve of the Cupid's bow. The eyes were abnormally small, were set wide apart, and appeared sunken into the face. He dreaded times like these. It had happened only twenty-five or so times in his career, but there was no easy way to handle it. Rousing from his silence, the professional of thirty years took over.

"This little guy seems to have some problems."

Stacey fought back hysteria. "What is it, Doctor?" She sobbed, exhausted physically and emotionally.

"Stacey, do you drink much?" Her prenatal history form revealed no alcohol intake, but Dr. Johnson knew that information was not always reliable.

"Only on weekends, and then not that much."

"Were you ever drunk during your pregnancy?"

She had a glass of wine on the weekend with friends, but never...

Suddenly, she remembered. The week with friends on a houseboat at Lake Powell, before she knew she was pregnant. They had drunk quite a bit. Her long silence accented the tomblike atmosphere of the delivery room.

"Well, I am no expert, Stacey, but I am concerned that this little guy may have some physical changes due to alcohol. We'll call Dr. Patterson to get his input. I'm sorry."

Dr. Albert Patterson, a noted expert in newborn retardation syndromes who taught at the university medical school, confirmed the diagnosis: baby boy Griffith suffered from fetal alcohol syndrome. For parents Tom and Stacey, a life of grief, disappointment, and hard work was about to begin.

Dustin Griffith was a "floppy" baby, a term given to infants with decreased muscle tone, which will later be reflected in poor muscle coordination. Dustin will not be shortstop on his local high school baseball team. In fact, in school he will require special education classes. His congenital neurological defects, brought on by alcohol in his mother's circulation while critical areas of his brain and nervous system were developing, will make him a lifelong challenge for his parents and for society. He will have a low IQ, poor memory, poor anger management, low academic ability, poor impulse control, and a severe form of attention deficit disorder. He will require special schooling all through his formative years, and only with extreme good fortune will he be able to be a productive member of society, working at a minimum wage job.

Most people think fetal alcohol syndrome occurs only in mothers who are hard-core alcoholics. Not so. Although it is true that severe fetal alcohol syndrome occurs in babies born to chronic alcoholics, growth retardation and fetal neurological deficits may be produced by maternal intake of as little as one drink (1.5 ounces of alcohol, 5 ounces of wine, 12 ounces of beer) a day. It has also been associated with "heavy episodic" drinking like Stacey's at the lake. And the effects are devastating.

The public is not aware of the great harm to individuals and the cost to society caused by maternal alcohol abuse. Startlingly, fetal alcohol syndrome (FAS) may account for up to 5 percent of all the mental retardation in the United States. Nine billion dollars annually is spent on individuals with fetal alcohol syndrome, devouring 11 percent of state and federal budgets for mental retardation. It is estimated that state and federal governments will spend up to 1.4 million dollars on a child with fetal alcohol syndrome in the course of his lifetime. Countless more children with subtle learning and attention deficit disorders may be the result of mild forms of fetal alcohol syndrome. Many such disorders do not produce the characteristic physical changes yet affect a child's school success and add to the burgeoning special education population, negatively impacting schools' budgets.

The American Academy of Pediatrics recommends a program of public education at the high school and college level to make young women aware that there is no "safe" amount of alcohol that can be consumed immediately before or during pregnancy. Complete abstinence from alcohol in women who are pregnant, or who are planning to get pregnant, is the only sure prevention.

But for Stacey and Tom Griffith, it is too late. Their lives will be forever altered by a week of binge drinking. Their future will not be filled with soccer games and chaperoning the prom. It will be filled with special education classes, medication, conferences with psychologists, and prayers that somehow their son might make it, if marginally, in adult society.

A terrible price for a week of partying.

DESECRATION

"Each second we live is a new and unique moment of the universe, a moment that never was before and will never be again. And what do we teach our children in school? We teach them that 2 and 2 makes 4 and that Paris is the capital of France. When will we also teach them what they are? We should say to each of them: Do you know what you are? You are a marvel. You are unique. In all the world there is no other child like you. And look at your body…what a wonder it is! Your legs, your arms, your cunning fingers, the way you move! You have the capacity for anything. Yes, you are a marvel. And when you grow up, can you harm another who is, like you, a marvel? You must cherish one another. You must work—we all must work—to make this world worthy of its children."

—Pablo Casals

How can we desecrate this unique and marvelous being that we are with an addictive chemical? How can we respond to God's perfect gift to us by poisoning our bodies and our souls?

The answer is simple. It's not a conscious, willful decision. It is an addiction.

12

MY LIFE WITH THE BOTTLE PART II

I carried a lot of emotional baggage as I made the transition from college to medical school. I had my amphetamine addiction, an uncertainty that I could handle the workload after four years of poor study habits, and a broken heart from a failed first serious relationship. From the start, I was in trouble. I went to class but just couldn't study at night. It was the educational equivalent of writer's block. But I had my supply of Eskatrol. My dental school chum had hooked me up with his doctor, and likewise I had been put on Dr. Wayne Callings's weight loss program, which included, of course, a prescription for Eskatrol.

Transitioning from undergraduate to medical school was a shock. I attended class eight hours a day, five days a week. I'd arrive home exhausted and stare at textbooks the size of telephone books, the language of which I couldn't begin to understand. When I tried to read one, I had to look up every third word in a medical dictionary. I was terrified. Like a deer in the headlights, I was paralyzed. Midterms rolled around and I pulled three all-nighters with my trusty Eskatrol. I learned the entire anatomy of the head and neck in one night. When I walked into the exam the next morning, I felt confident. But as I read each question, it seemed that at least two answers of the five multiples were correct. Which one was more correct? I skipped to the next question, only to find the same scenario. When I finished the exam, I had answered only eighteen of the sixty questions. Panic began to creep in as I went back through, trying to divine which of the two correct answers was more correct. I looked at my watch. There was only ten minutes left. The faster I tried to go, the more panicked I became. Finally, the bell rang. I had left ten questions unanswered. I bombed the exam, barely making a passing grade.

That anatomy exam set the tone for the entire year. I was so fearful of studying that I couldn't, I didn't. I crammed in a hyperintense atmosphere and then choked on the exams. School, my personal life, and the speed combined to create a nightmare of fear and dread. I finished the year sixtieth in a class of sixty-four. I was miserable. The worst aspect of my dependence on Eskatrol was coming down from four days straight on the drug. There was a rebound of exhaustion and depression that was almost unbearable, coupled with physical pain as the drug cleared my system.

I was not the only drug user in the freshman class. Half my classmates were taking speed to study. Most fared better than I. Several did not. One unlucky classmate, a pharmacological adventurer who shared a cadaver with me in anatomy, fried his brain on the last day of finals and wrote an entire ten-page blue book, ironically on psychiatric disorders, on the first page of the book, writing each page over the preceding one. The page was illegible and he failed the exam, that class, and several others and was asked to repeat the year. He did and prospers as a psychiatrist somewhere in the affluence and neuroses of southern California.

The end of my freshman year brought an honest appraisal and reevaluation of the direction my life had taken. I knew I could not continue my chemical roller coaster. I wouldn't survive. I had the summer to find an exit strategy. By some miracle, I learned of a summer research fellowship in neurosurgery with a world-renowned doctor in the field and was accepted. Unknowingly, I was about to forge a relationship that would change my life. Robert H. Pudenz, MD, who had recently lost his son to suicide, would heal my wounds of fear and self-doubt as I healed his profound grief. Dr. Pudenz believed in me completely and taught me to believe in myself. The work I did with him that and the following summer was some of the finest I have ever done. I began the new academic year resolved that I would never take drugs to study, even if it meant failing out, and I was good to my word. I earned straight A's that second year and went from sixtieth to sixteenth in my class, and my life completely turned around. I recognized that I had been addicted to speed and that I had some characteristics of an addictive personality. Sadly, I didn't recognize that I had the same problem with alcohol, only a less severe, less obvious, and seemingly more harmless one. I didn't drink any more than most of my friends did, certainly a lot less than my parents and a lot less than I had in the fraternity. But alcohol was an intimate friend, something I enjoyed, looked forward to, needed. I might have been a long way upstream, but I was in the current headed for the rapids above a deadly waterfall. It would take thirty years to get to the brink and the necessity to swim for my life. Thank God

I made it. How unfortunate that I couldn't learn the lesson when I was in medical school.

You may be thinking, "He's overreacting. He didn't really have a problem. He functioned well. Maybe he needed a drink now and then to relax or unwind, but he wasn't an alcoholic." That may be true for some people, but it wasn't true for me. I now know that I drank alcohol for the chemical effect that it had on me, just as I took Eskatrol to study. I was developing a physiological and social need for alcohol, although it was barely recognizable for many years. But that's the way alcohol is. You drink it seemingly harmlessly for many years and then, one day, if you are lucky, you wake up to the fact that it has changed you. It changed me: I was a different person when I drank. It changed my personality. I was more skeptical, cynical, mistrusting, angry, and at times downright mean. And after many years, I realized that alcohol could really make me depressed. I was using alcohol out of habit but also because I thought it helped me cope with anxiety, stress, and depression. It doesn't. It is a poor drug for all three and it can increase depression as it did for me. I finally quit because I didn't like the person I was when I drank. I didn't like what my friends became when they drank. Now, my feelings and the person that I am are both real. I am not altered by alcohol. And I genuinely like myself sober a lot more.

Another of my addictive behaviors was smoking. I began the day I moved into the dorms my freshman year of college and continued through the middle of my second year of medical school. I was really something, pulling those all-nighters my first year in med school, drinking Diet Coke or coffee, puffing away on a cigarette, and reading a textbook. I remember the second quarter of my freshman year I smoked so heavily the last night of finals that I burned the roof of my mouth. It sloughed out in one thick leathery piece two days later. I was subconsciously disgusted but laughed about it to all my friends. I considered it a necessary evil to help me get through school.

In the second quarter of my sophomore year in med school, after I had successfully given up speed, I did my very first physical examination on a patient as a student doctor. The patient was dying of end-stage emphysema, and I was shocked at the cruelty of that disease. He had been a steelworker, helping to build some of the high-rise buildings that dotted the Los Angeles skyline. In his prime, he was 230 pounds, standing six feet two. He weighed 116 pounds when I examined him, a skin-covered skeleton. He panted like a wheezing steam engine, trying to deliver precious oxygen to lungs that couldn't absorb it. He was so short of breath that he couldn't close his mouth to chew a bite of food, and he could only answer my questions in monosyllables.

I had never seen emphysema up close. After several prior failed attempts to quit smoking, I took an intimate look at the ravages of this disease and never smoked again. This was the third example of the addictive nature of my personality, but I never connected my prior addictions to speed and tobacco with my use of alcohol. I saw myself as a social drinker, like all my friends, and certainly no more than that. It was the norm to drink on the weekends and at parties, and it was okay to get a little tipsy on occasion. It is fascinating to reflect back now that I didn't know any nondrinkers. There was no one around to question the premise, nothing to alter the behavior. Nothing to challenge the denial.

In medical school and in residency, my finances and social status allowed me to begin to drink hard liquor. The beer and cheap wine gave way to distilled spirits and good wine. I tried gin and tonics, vodka and tonics, and bourbon and seven, and I settled on Scotch and water. My wife and I took some wine-tasting classes and joined a club with several other residents in my training program. We read books, sampled, and began to develop a taste for fine wines. Well on the way to becoming wine snobs, we bought some good wine to put away and rented a locker at a local liquor store that was temperature- and humidity-controlled to store our considerable investment.

I quit the hard stuff after Joe got me sick on it. Several years into my residency, it came about as the result of a dinner at my in-laws' house. Joe, my father-in-law, was the quintessential salesman, possessing a toothy smile and a hearty handshake. We dined with them one evening after I had spent several consecutive near all-nighters staffing an emergency room. I was fuzzy with fatigue and his scotch tasted good. Joe was not one to skimp on the alcohol, and he made sure my glass was refilled promptly. After three or four scotch and waters that were mostly scotch, I was pretty drunk. My wife drove home. I was very sick, but borrowing a page from my college days, I unloaded as much of the dinner and the alcohol as I could as soon as we got home. From a very early age, I've excelled at self-induced vomiting. As a kid, I developed horrendous headaches from eating pork. Eventually, it would make me vomit, and as soon as I did, my headache disappeared. As a result, I learned to gag myself with my finger and induce retching. It came in handy during my college years and it helped that night when Joe plied me with scotch. Despite relieving myself of probably half the scotch, I still felt awful the next day. I made my wife promise she wouldn't let on to her dad. I felt bad enough and didn't want to give Joe the satisfaction of knowing how ill I had been. After that, I lost my taste for scotch and gave up other distilled spirits.

The alcohol content was too high. It was possible to drink too much too fast and get way beyond a controllable level of intoxication. I would drink wine with meals, and a margarita or fancy rum concoction on occasion, but as time went on I became almost exclusively a beer drinker. I love the taste of beer, and with its relatively low alcohol content, I could drink quite a bit without getting drunk. And if I did start feeling drunk, I could ease up and control the level of intoxication much more easily than I could when drinking hard liquor. I never rationalized that I wasn't drinking that much. I knew and agreed with the old adage "If you drink a lot of beer, you drink a lot." But it was a more user-friendly vehicle that fit my lifestyle and I liked the taste.

After I quit smoking, I took up another addiction. I began to run. Running is more than an activity that produces fitness. It is a passion that can become an addiction. I was aware of that at some level, but I rationalized that it was a healthy addiction. I ran out of resolve to control a lifelong weight problem and to mitigate the stress of medical school and the emotional intensity that studying produced. After three or four hours of studying, usually with several cups of coffee, an hour-long run would relax me, allow my racing mind to slow down, and permit precious sleep.

I ran for five years on my own—for exercise, for fitness, and as a stress releaser. I began with a mile a day, then three, and after five years, I was running six miles a day with an occasional ten-mile run on the weekend. Then one day another runner pulled up on my shoulder, complimented my pace, and invited me to his running club's half-marathon the next day. I didn't think much of my ability and I was intimidated by the idea of running against others in competition. But curiosity got the better of me and I showed up the next day and ran the half-marathon (13.1 miles) in eighty-one minutes. That finished me well up in the pack and earned the congratulations of many of the club's runners. Realizing that my time was well under the pace required to achieve the sub-three-hour qualification to run the Boston Marathon, I was hooked. I made the abrupt transition from recreational runner to serious running junkie.

Running and beer drinking are practically synonymous. The beverage of choice after a long hot training run is an ice-cold lager or two or five. I used to joke that running was an excuse to drink beer, and it was partially true. Some of the best fellowship I have ever experienced was sitting on the lawn after a hard run and drinking a six-pack or two with a bunch of running buddies. There was camaraderie and a commonness of purpose that was intimate and very satisfying. Runners are a great group. Intensely fit, they value physical effort and discipline, and unlike my often-arrogant physician acquaintances, they come from every walk of life. I was good enough, just barely, to be one of them. Within this circle there was a broad spectrum of running abilities: from college cross-country medalists to fitness runners. An amiable and gregarious group, they all shared the love of running and of beer.

Running fulfilled a great many of my needs. I had always struggled with a weight problem, and running allowed me to control it. When I first started in the early 1970s, I developed a running variant of anorexia nervosa. During my quarter of med school in England, I went more than a little bit overboard on the running. British school didn't start until 9 AM, so I ran ten miles each morning before school. I ate only one meal a day, dinner, and I controlled my hunger the rest of the time by eating fresh carrots. I'm just shy of six feet two, and in my chubby days early in med school, I weighed just over 200. When I came back from England, I weighed 158. I looked a bit gaunt and had an orange cast to my skin from all the beta-carotene (it's a very good internal sunscreen and free radical quencher, but that's another story). It took a year for me to recover from the anorexia, to correct my skewed perception of my body image, and to fill out a little. But running, at the level I chose to do it, always allowed me to eat (and drink) anything I wanted without getting back to my pre-running weight.

Running also gave me a lot of confidence. The discipline required generalized into other areas of my life. I was never as focused and as happy as when I was training for a marathon or other big race.

I also experienced the running "high" a lot. When I was really fit, I felt an intense sense of well-being almost every day. Running is one of nature's antidepressants. The only downside was that I could drink as much as I wanted and not get fat *or* feel the depression that occurs when people drink heavily. So insight and awareness of the negative effects of alcohol would await a time when I couldn't continue running.

I ran for thirty years. Hard. I averaged between fifty and seventy miles a week. Through it all, beer was my training partner. Only once did we part company. In the late 1980s, I was training for a hundred-mile run. As part of my Spartan discipline, I gave up alcohol for the last two months before the race. I remember feeling intensely well, but I thought it was my physical shape. After finishing the race, I drank a quart of Budweiser, savoring the taste. Later, I remember wistfully thinking I wished I had continued my sobriety, but it was too late. I was drinking again.

One of the problems with my personality, my physical needs, and my chemical makeup is that I can't just drink one beer. I begin to feel that mellowness, and

I want another, and another. For me it's all or nothing. So, now for me it's nothing.

If my knees hadn't begun to wear out, I may never have developed the insight I needed to quit drinking. After five arthroscopic surgeries, I finally had to accept the inevitability that I couldn't run at my previous level of intensity. Gone was the "endorphin high." Gone was the antidepressant. But the beer kept flowing. The result was a bulging middle, and a hard-to-pinpoint depression that I attributed to not being able to run, reaching middle age (a dubious accomplishment), and the stresses of an intensely busy medical practice. It took a long while for me to realize it was the alcohol.

But today, five years into my sobriety, the depression is gone. It is wonderful to know that the feelings I experience are real and not induced by a chemical I've ingested. I have defeated four addictive behaviors in my fifty-plus years: nail biting, smoking, amphetamines, and alcohol. Alcohol was definitely the hardest. The crux of the problem was denial because I had been raised in a family of high-functioning alcoholics and didn't know what "normal" was. Denial because I had never missed a day of school or work as a result of my drinking, which I thought was an important criterion for a problem drinker. Denial because I had seen "real" alcoholics in the admitting ward at County Hospital, and I was nothing like those people. Denial because all my friends drank as much or more than I did. I had no point of reference for nondrinking. Denial in thinking that the addictive personality that had trouble with speed and tobacco would not have trouble with alcohol.

13

DOCTORS MAKE GREAT ALCOHOLICS AND DRUG ADDICTS

His palms were covered with thick scales that were cracked, fissured, and painful, caused by such severe psoriasis that he couldn't use his hands. Roger was one of three principal operators of the Diablo Nuclear Power Plant on the rocky coast near our town. In those hands rested the safety of literally millions.

Miraculously, one of the lesser-known drugs for psoriasis, initially developed to treat malaria and leprosy, cleared up Roger's hands. For twelve years, his hands had been normal and his job secure. In spite of that, the psoriasis on the rest of his body worsened. Large, beefy red, scaly plaques covered his forearms and shins. It would just be a while before his hands were unusable again. Perhaps it was time for a change, but the other powerful drugs for psoriasis all had the side effect of liver toxicity.

"Roger, do you drink much?"

"Not at all, Doc."

My medical training and the experience of being lied to and disappointed by countless patients left me a little skeptical. I pursued.

"Not at all?"

"No."

"Why not?"

"My dad was an ophthalmologist, and he was a drunk."

"Really?"

"Yeah. And when I drank as a young man, I could always see myself becoming like him. So, I quit."

"Did you have a problem with it?"

"I could have. I didn't let it go that far."

"Did you go the AA route?"

"No, I just quit."

"What were you like when you drank?"

"I talked too much. It changed me."

"Did it make you mean?"

"No, just different. Alcohol just changes people. They're not the same."

"Your dad was an ophthalmologist?"

"Yeah. And he was drunk every night. He would get argumentative."

"You kept your head down at dinner and left as soon as you finished eating because he wanted to pick a fight?" I had lived through a lot of the same family meals.

"Lots of times, I wouldn't go to dinner. I would lie that I had to study and I would eat in my room and leave him to my brother and my poor mom."

"And she just put up with it?"

"Yeah. What else was she going to do? He was her meal ticket. Besides, lots of people were like that then."

"Still are, but we tolerate it less."

Roger's dad was a high-functioning alcoholic. He was a highly successful and respected ophthalmologist. But he drank three double martinis every night, and he died of alcoholic cirrhosis at seventy-three. His children and wife, who had suffered so much punishment over the years, did not mourn much.

Doctors make great drug abusers, especially of alcohol. I don't distinguish between drug abuse and alcoholism because alcohol is a drug. Alcohol is socially accepted, so we don't think of it in the same sense as heroin or speed or cocaine, but it is no different. My recovering drug abusers from the Liberty Tattoo Program taught me that. A drug is a drug.

There are several reasons why doctors make great drug abusers. First, many are more than a little bit obsessive-compulsive. They had to be to get through medical school and residency. Where discipline ends and obsessive-compulsive behavior begins is a fine line that many medical students cross over. That obsessive-compulsive nature is fertile ground for addiction.

Second, they have easy access to all kinds of drugs. Whether in the medication cupboard on the hospital ward or the sample cabinet in his office, the physician has ready access to pain medication, mood-altering drugs, and sleeping pills. Salespersons from various drug companies are constantly plying doctors with the newest and latest medications and giving them free samples to try on their patients (or themselves). When I was an intern at LA County-USC Medical Center, we were still using liquid cocaine to anesthetize noses in the ear, nose, and throat emergency room. The hospital eventually had to change anesthetics because the cocaine would mysteriously disappear on an almost daily basis.

Third, physicians are under enormous amounts of stress. Caring for sick people is a very hard job. The decision making required to diagnose and treat serious illness is daunting. Enormous anxiety results from the fear of making the wrong decision, which may result in a patient's worsening or dying (renamed in current spin parlance as "a negative patient outcome"). Often, with attorneys breathing down their necks, anxiety may also produce a negative emotional and financial outcome for doctors.

Last, doctors almost universally have huge egos and are supremely confident that "they can handle it." Overconfident, with an inflated sense of self, they believe they have the willpower and the personal power to overcome any potential problems, any risk of addiction. That's why they are such poor pilots. With overinflated self-worth, they cannot conceive encountering an unsolvable problem in the air. So they fly in marginal weather, take risks, and "know" they can't run out of gas. But statistics show they are, as a group, the most likely to be involved in fatal crashes. The self-assuredness that creates good physicians and inspires confidence in patients makes them poor pilots. It also makes them vulnerable to alcohol and other drug addictions.

Historically, one of the best examples of physicians' vulnerability to drug addiction is William Halstead. Halstead was a world-famous surgeon, certainly the greatest American doctor of his generation. He was the chief surgeon at Johns Hopkins College of Medicine in Baltimore. He was brilliant, innovative, and dedicated. Many of the surgical procedures and instruments for general surgery still bear his name.

Halstead also discovered the efficacy of cocaine as a local anesthetic. Traveling in South America, he noticed the natives chewing the leaves of the coca plant as they toiled long hours in the hot tropical sun. They seemed to have boundless energy, and on occasion, he noticed individuals who accidentally became injured and marveled that they seemed insensitive to the pain of the injury. Halstead began experimenting with an extract of the leaves and found that it was a superb local anesthetic, used both topically or injected. As so many physicians did in the early days of modern medicine, he experimented on himself and, in the process, became hopelessly addicted to cocaine. A nineteenth-century detox program, a sailing trip to the Windward Islands, was arranged. Halstead recovered. He returned to a normal life for several years but became addicted again later in his life and died a cocaine and morphine addict.

George Walker was a good old boy from Tennessee, a fine surgeon who drank too much. He never drank during the day, but in the evening he'd have two or three tall glasses of Tennessee-sipping whiskey. It started innocently enough as social drinking, acceptable at the time, but as the years passed, his dependence became stronger, the need was greater, and the quantity increased. As happens to so many high-functioning alcoholics, the vortex of the disease trapped George, and he was sucked in.

There were several occasions when he was called in to the emergency room to see patients in the evening and observant nurses smelled alcohol on his breath. One night, while examining a ten-year-old girl with appendicitis, he was unsteady and slurring his words. Amazingly enough he operated on her, and she recovered uneventfully; however, the potential for disaster loomed in the operating room. An unsteady hand could nick the bowel, leading to a fatal peritonitis, or an altered judgment could fail to see a small artery that retracted up into the mesentery, causing the patient to hemorrhage after surgery.

Hospitals and their staffs run like the military. Years ago nurses would never dare to question a doctor's judgment or physical condition. George's inebriation continued for quite some time until one of the nurses had the courage to say something to another doctor. Once alerted, the doctor made a point of observing George a time or two in the ER after dark. In keeping with the good old boy network of doctors, Walker was not reported and referred for therapy. Instead the chief of surgery mentioned to George at their weekly golf game that alcohol on his breath had been noticed in the ER and he had better be more careful. Also, Walker's partners covered for him, telling the ER staff not to call him in the evening unless they couldn't get in touch with anyone else.

This continued for years. After he retired, his drinking increased and contributed to high blood pressure and a stroke, which killed George in his late sixties. It is amazing how long a person can live with a serious alcohol problem.

Why didn't his wife intervene during his years of alcoholism? Since she was not a drinker, her husband's alcoholic intake must have been painfully clear. Her unwillingness to address this issue could have stemmed from loyalty to her spouse or from fear of a radical change in lifestyle if he was discovered, had to go to rehab, or lost his license. The shame and disgrace of admitting to and dealing with the problem and the traditional mentality of covering up one's dirty laundry and standing by your man possibly prevented her from acting. It contributed to several decades of worsening addiction, jeopardy to countless patients, and the eventual death of a fine man and a good surgeon.

Alcoholism still has a social stigma. Our present attitudes toward alcohol are reminiscent of societal views of mental illness a half a century ago, which espoused that it was a genetic weakness in your family tree never to be revealed. Today, with increased understanding and public education, it is understood that many of these diseases are chemical imbalances or genetic abnormalities to identify and treat. The same must occur with alcoholism. It is a disease, not a character weakness. It needs to be diagnosed without any social innuendo. And once diagnosed, treatment is very effective. Abstention immediately begins to reverse most of the physical and psychiatric damage. Psychotherapy and a twelve-step program usually facilitate insight into the problem, which, along with behavior modification, greatly reduces the chance of relapse.

The medical profession is beginning to see the light. A program now exists in which addicted physicians can enter rehabilitation programs and not lose their licenses. An anonymous hotline is available to report the "impaired physician," leading to earlier identification of addicted doctors. The initial motivation may have been fear of liability, but the benefit to patient welfare and safety has become apparent since the advent of the program.

In spite of that, the quarterly bulletin of the California Board of Medical Quality Assurance (BOMQUA) lists twenty to thirty doctors whose licenses have been suspended or revoked due to drug and alcohol abuse. And that's just the tip of the iceberg.

Physicians are bright, and many with addictive problems are very clever and more than a little devious. Take, for instance, Ken Porter. Ken was a year ahead of me in medical school and close friends with a buddy of mine, Tom Downing. As Tom tells it, the very first day of medical school this big handsome guy stuck a huge ham of a hand out at his, and from that day on, they were fast friends. He seemed like the nicest guy in the whole world. Later, as Tom began to see Ken's dark side, he was never sure if it had always existed and he had been deceived from the beginning, or if the drugs and alcohol had gradually eroded Ken's morality. They studied together, he on his Eskatrol and Tom on his. Ken also worked a lot. He was married in his first year and had a child by the summer before his second. Attending medical school with a wife and a child on meager funds was tough. Ken needed to work to supplement his grants and loans. When he was a fourth-year student, our hospital was short of interns on Obstetrics and Gynecology, so they hired fourth-year students to work as interns. Tom worked one night a week. Ken worked two in addition to the time demands of his fourth year. Tom was always amazed at Ken's energy level. As he looks back on it, it was probably pharmacologically induced.

Ken chose internal medicine as a specialty and remained at Los Angeles County. The hours were long and the work hard. Ken was incredible. He was never tired, never down. Occasionally the three of us met socially and drank Rusty Nails together (a mixture of scotch and Drambuie). Whenever I saw him, I marveled at his stamina and enthusiasm. Everyone I know felt the same about Ken.

When something seems too good to be true, it generally is. Ken was probably taking drugs then to maintain the killer pace of his life.

Ken moved with his wife and now growing family to the Central Coast a year ahead of me. He actually arranged an interview for me at the clinic where he had taken a job, and his presence in the area was a huge inducement for me to come. After I arrived, we saw less of each other than we had before. I dismissed it as his busy life and a little jealousy on his wife's part. I now realize Ken had parts of his life he didn't want me to see. He worked a killer schedule under the guise of providing for a large and growing family, but he had Mercedes tastes and he liked to indulge them.

I started having some doubts about Ken when he mentioned that he had his wife on powerful antidepressants. One of the cardinal rules in medicine is that physicians ethically should not treat themselves or their families, as it clouds their judgment and it is taboo. Why would Ken choose to diagnose and treat his wife? Why was she depressed?

Then, Ken left his clinic under a cloud of controversy. His contract provided that all his income would be shared with the group, yet he had been doing a lot of outside consulting and keeping the money. Ken believed that he was practically supporting the clinic with his office income and they had no right to any more. The clinic stated that Ken breached his contract.

Being the good friend, I helped Ken move his desk and files out of the clinic on a weekend, before they had a chance to lock him out. He was my friend and I supported him. I did not suspect that his drug use might be eroding his ethical judgment.

After Ken left the clinic, he opened his own office and his practice flourished. To this day, ten years later, patients we had in common will tell you that he was the best doctor they ever had. And he was. But he left his wife for a nurse he met at the hospital, and many rumors circulated that it was not the first. Or even the tenth.

The divorce settlement of the decade was followed by a few more years of practice and then, suddenly, Ken left town. He said he was frustrated with the medical climate in California, the low reimbursement of Medicare, and the

HMOs and would relocate in Oklahoma where a doctor could still make a good living. I heard that he was being investigated for billing irregularities and might be restricted by some insurance companies from seeing their patients. Whatever the case, he is gone and owns his own clinic and hospital in rural Oklahoma.

He deserted his staff with a suddenness that was startling. Employees of two decades were left without a job or any retirement provision. One of his nurses came in to see me a while back and was still in shock at the way she had been treated. Without rancor she recounted how she gradually discovered that Ken had a drug abuse problem. She finally confronted him with it and threatened to turn him in. He was more careful about not letting her see his problem until he finally left town.

I asked how he managed to do it. She said he was masterful at regulating his level of consciousness. When he was tired, he took uppers; when he was wired, he took downers. The right drug for the right mood.

Can people do that for a lifetime? Maybe. Maybe he'll get away with it. Or perhaps he'll end up like Eric Cavanaugh.

Eric was a brilliant man, one of the smartest men I ever met. He was multitalented: a fine athlete with a keen mind and shrewd business savvy. Like Roger Tate's dad, Eric was an ophthalmologist. He trained at the best schools, and by all accounts, he had excellent clinical judgment when it came to patients.

But he had a drinking problem and a drug problem. Eric was one of those people to whom everything came too easily. He was the kind of student that never had to study and aced the tests anyway. Eric would quickly master a subject or a sport and then become bored. He was always looking for the next challenge, the next adrenaline rush. In research science or some field of inquiry with unlimited questions, and the right direction, Eric could have been a great scientist, a Nobel Prize winner. But his prime motivation was money and status, and he had a fatal flaw: he believed he could drink and experiment with drugs and not get burned.

There's no telling when the serious problems began. When I met him he was sixty and he had clearly been compromised for at least a decade. He drank every evening. Hard. His adult children refused to have dinner with him or to stop by in the evening because he got drunk and ugly. But he also self-medicated with uppers and downers and whatever was the latest psychoactive drug on the market. He mixed and matched. The arrogant are particularly subject to the seduction of drugs and alcohol because they think they are too smart to get into trouble. They'll recognize a problem developing and are strong enough to overcome the addiction. It's not going to happen to them.

Wrong. Drugs and alcohol are great equalizers. They do not discriminate between the rich and the poor or between the smart and the not so keen. They will addict all with the same fierce grip.

Almost imperceptibly, Eric began to slip: a bill unpaid here, a critical clause in a contract not read there, a flawed business decision made now that never would have occurred ten years before. And, there were moments of confusion. Eric would awaken at night, confused at his surroundings. He was subject to dreadful nightmares. Within five years Eric gradually spiraled into profound dementia. As of this writing, he is in a locked facility and doesn't recognize his wife or children. He has coarse tremors and a wide-based, staggering gate, and he is deteriorating rapidly. There is no other family history of dementia.

What happens to brain cells that are so radically altered by alcohol and psychoactive drugs? Critical brain chemicals, the neurotransmitters, are produced in greater or lesser amounts and become depleted in some areas of the brain. The normal release and reuptake is changed, forever. This system is very complex and in delicate balance, and our emotional and mental health is completely dependent on it. Awareness must be increased that drinking and doing drugs negatively alter this necessary balance.

In England, alcoholism is institutionalized in medicine. I had the good fortune of spending my senior summer in medical school in London, studying pathology at Westminster Hospital. As I have previously related, I had drunk my share in college and I thought I could hold my own at the bar. The Brits, however, took it to a new level.

I arrived in early summer. That week, the Rugby Club held its annual banquet and I was invited to attend. Since I felt a little self-conscious and unfamiliar, I declined the banquet but agreed to arrive later for the after-dinner party. I was a little early, in time to hear the featured speaker, Sir Geoffrey Organe, physician to the queen, speak on "The Importance of the Kick" in rugby. As the group seemed a little rowdy after several hours of imbibing, I wondered how such a serious talk would be received. I soon found out. Within several minutes of beginning his dissertation, Sir Geoffrey, adorned in black tie and tails with medals of his rank in British Society, was pelted with dinner rolls and strawberries.

"Aw, piss off, Sir Geoffrey," was the refrain from the inebriated athletes. Embarrassed for the stately gentleman, I retreated to the bar (yes, there was a bar in the medical school) and sipped a pint of bitter. The banquet soon broke up and the party moved to the bar, where some already sloppy medical students and housemen (interns and residents) tried to carry a tune as they regaled me with traditional and bawdy rugby songs. They drank nothing but beer, but they drank a lot of it, and the party became increasingly raucous. Among new friends, I was on my best behavior and drinking very little. I was astounded at how much these Brits could drink and how soluble the stiff English reserve was with a couple of pints. There were housemen drinking in the bar who were "on call" at the hospital, which adjoined the medical school. Even then, my sense of medical ethics was offended. The evening ended with forty-odd medical students carrying the piano from the bar out onto the sidewalk along Vauxhall Bridge Road, chopping it up with an ax, and lighting it on fire. Passersby in vehicles were stopped and handed a pint for their perilous journey across the Thames, until the glasses ran out.

I thought this alcoholic near-anarchy was perhaps a once-a-year meltdown of the usually reserved British medical students, tolerated by the authorities because of its infrequent occurrence. But when a similar but slightly less destructive gathering was held the following week, I came to understand that this kind of behavior is acceptable, perhaps even expected.

The next event, a bachelor party for the president of the Rugby Club, was held the night before his wedding, in one of the apartments of the medical students. The beer flowed freely and there were a lot of walking wounded by the end of the evening. The "call of the moose" could be heard frequently from the loo as many of the students recalled their dinners and earlier refreshments. In the end, the president passed out cold as a mackerel. Those still standing dragged him down to "Casualty," the British equivalent of our emergency room, had him fitted with a spica cast (a full-body jacket in plaster), and put him on a bus for Manchester, five hundred miles away. No one seemed worried that he might vomit, aspirate the vomitus down his lungs, and develop an oftentimes fatal aspiration pneumonia. By some miracle, he survived and even made it back for the wedding, though he looked a little peaked.

Just a little harmless fun? Hardly. A college or university student dies of alcohol poisoning once a week in the UK, and by sanctioning and institutionalizing alcohol abuse, they are recruiting young people who otherwise might not drink and opening the door to the possibility of future alcoholism.

American medical students and young doctors are no better. When I was an intern in 1972, I lived in a twelve-story dormitory for interns at LA County-USC Medical Center. The lower ten floors were for single interns, the upper two for married. Still hung over from the drug craze of the turbulent sixties, the dorms were a hotbed of alcohol and drug abuse. The ringleader was a tall, gangly intern from New Jersey named Mark Roth. Coming from the big city, Mark was more worldly and pharmaceutically wise than his provincial California colleagues and he led the way in chemical exploration for many young interns. And it always began with alcohol.

Mark had his one-room studio in the dorms decorated like an opium den. A large Persian carpet hung suspended from the ceiling only six inches above head level. The walls were covered with aluminum foil, and the state-of-the-art stereo was wired to colored lights and strobes. A large multifaceted glass orb slowly rotated from the center of the ceiling, just at head level.

Mark had parties. Lots of parties. He was homozygous for the lazy gene and was masterful at trading the more difficult one-month rotations away for leisurely months on psychiatry or neurology, which had very little call. This allowed more entertaining.

I chose some difficult elective rotations and retained the killer months on Medicine, so during my small snatches of free time, I tried to get caught up on my sleep or spent it with my wife. I did, however, attend one party at Mark's. It was the last night of our internship. I was IOC (intern on call: a roving intern summoned to any of the medical wards to restart IVs, de-impact petrified colons, or pronounce patients dead), so I couldn't drink, but I wanted to observe the goings-on.

It was amazing. Psychedelic music blared, lights flashed, beer tabs popped among bodies crammed in so tight you couldn't move, with a thick haze of marijuana smoke hanging from the Persian carpet to shoulder height so you couldn't even identify the person standing beside you. I refused several joints as they circulated around the room, sipped a Diet Coke, and took it all in.

A hash pipe passed by. The bathroom door was opened a crack, revealing surreptitious activity and furtive looks. They were snorting cocaine.

I was called to the hospital to restart an IV. When I returned, there were huge cartons of ice cream, a dozen different flavors, circulating, each with several large spoons stuck in them. The leading doctors of the next generation were completely drunk and stoned. And for some, the road ahead would be bumpy, replete with alcoholism and multiple drug use that ended in tragedy.

Mark got busted ten years later. His license was suspended but the suspension was stayed. He spent two years in a diversion program, but by all accounts, he's still abusing. He knows he's smarter than the law and believes he's just a recreational user. Two more of my fellow interns appeared in the medical board's quarterly journal: license revoked for self-prescribing; license suspended for drug and alcohol abuse.

GARMAN, JOHN A., M.D. (A32107) Downey, CA
B & P Code SS2234 (e), 2236 (a), 2239 (a), 2261.
Arrested twice for driving under the influence and received one conviction for reckless driving (author's note: This is a "wet reckless" as explained in chapter 31), failed to report either arrest to his Board probation monitor, made false statements in an application for reappointment as a qualified medical examiner, and violated the terms and conditions of his Board-ordered probation. Revoked (his license). April 10, 2003.
From the quarterly report of the Medical Board of California.
(John Garman was a fraternity brother in college and several years ahead of me in medical school.)

It is frightening to think that the people we trust with our lives may be practicing under the influence, but some certainly are. The pressures of the job create enormous stress, and the long hours leave many physicians on the edge of exhaustion. The temptation to drink to relax or to take a pill to be more alert is enticing. And some succumb to it. Gradually, it becomes a pattern and then a habit, and for some it results in addiction. Some recover but many live enslaved by drugs and alcohol, and the profession they strove so hard to enter becomes a nightmare of deception and delusion.

14

SCOTT

My friend Scott died last night. A self-destructive force that he set in motion twenty-five years ago, a squamous cell cancer, finally had its way.

He grew up a good kid and talented athlete in Santa Cruz, California. Never a gifted student, he drifted toward manual skills in high school: wood shop, metal shop, and auto shop. There was no hint of the tragedy to come.

Unfortunately, he chose the wrong friends in high school. They drank beer and he joined in. He stopped attending church and drifted away from his family and their values. Scott progressed from beer to cocaine, and as so often happens, the alcohol and drugs consumed him. He borrowed money from drug dealers, who take a dim view of addicts who skip out on their debts. He stole from his parents, abandoning his sense of right to the demands of his addiction. Finally, with a warrant out for his arrest and some unsavory characters looking for him, Scott cowered in a flophouse closet contemplating suicide. In desperation, he called home instead. His dad would speak with him only at their pastor's house. When he arrived, the ultimatum given was detox or jail.

Scott spent a month in an inpatient recovery center in Monterey. That's where, on his first day, he met our mutual friend, Bud (chapter 22). Just out of D.T.s, Bud was trying to negotiate his way down the hall, but, still heavily medicated, he needed the wall for balance. Scott remembers seeing this disheveled person "sliding" along a wall coming toward him, never dreaming that they would become lifelong friends. They roomed together and have been soul and accountability friends ever since. As Bud likes to put it, Scott was "present at the creation."

Scott was one of the lucky ones, an addict who didn't die. Of the thirty people at the recovery center with Bud and Scott, only five are still alive. The rest succumbed to their recurrent addictions or committed suicide, attributable to the hopelessness of their failed attempts to remain clean and sober. Scott succeeded in his recovery and built a wonderful life. He married Peggy, channeled his obsessive nature into a passion for fishing, and worked as a building contractor known for his honesty and excellent product. He accomplished this through a reborn faith and continued participation in a twelve-step program.

The goal of recovery is not sobriety. It is contentment. Many recovering alcoholics are sober but they don't progress past abstinence to the attainment of peace. These "dry drunks" haven't faced and solved the many personal issues that fueled their addiction. They are simply abstinent. Scott progressed beyond sober to content. He was a genuinely happy person and had a wonderful sense of humor with clever perceptions that only enlighten a soul who has traveled to perdition and back. I am so privileged to have known Scott and to have shared his insights into drug and alcohol abuse. It's ironic that I was acquainted with Scott for several years before his illness but didn't really get to know him until he got sick. Coincidentally, that was just before I gave up drinking. Until I was sober, I was more than a little intimidated by his resolve. Only someone with the problem can appreciate the strength of someone in recovery. Once I was sober, I felt perfectly comfortable being with and getting to know Scott. It was a remarkable experience.

Unfortunately, the seeds of self-destruction sown during Scott's dark time reaped a harvest of cancer. Ten years of heavy drinking and smoking took a toll. Once a person sets in motion a destructive force, even if only subconsciously, and it progresses beyond a certain point, say to the development of a virulent cancer, it cannot be recalled. So it was with Scott. Three years ago, he came in for a checkup and showed me a lump on the right side of his neck which he had noticed a week before. It was firm but not rock-hard, and I thought it might simply be an enlarged lymph node from a prior sore throat. When it didn't diminish in two weeks on antibiotics, I referred him to an ear, nose, and throat specialist for a needle biopsy. It was inconclusive but suspicious for malignancy. What followed was an excisional biopsy, where the entire lump was removed and immediately examined with frozen sections. It turned out to be squamous cell cancer, metastatic to a lymph node in Scott's neck. As a result, at the time of the biopsy, Scott had a radical neck dissection, a ghastly procedure where all the lymph nodes and the major muscles of the left side of his neck were removed. At the same time, his mouth, throat, larynx, upper bronchi, and esophagus were examined with an endoscope and fifteen small biopsies were taken from any unusual-looking areas, in an attempt to find the primary cancer site. The final results showed cancer in three of the neck nodes but no definitely positive site that could be called the primary site. As you have already learned, the combination of heavy drinking and smoking are prime causes of squamous cancer of all the areas suspected of harboring Scott's primary.

Following the surgery, Scott had intense radiation to his neck and upper chest for six weeks, causing his throat to become so sore that he couldn't eat. A feeding tube was placed through his upper abdomen into his stomach that remained for three months after the treatments ended. He lost thirty pounds and never recovered his sense of taste or salivary gland function. He lived with a bottle of water in one hand and sipped on it constantly to moisten his radiation-burned mouth and throat.

There was a six-month period of relatively good health. Scott got back to work, and his days off and weekends reaped a rich harvest of salmon, halibut, and sea bass. He was happy, and with each passing day it looked as if he might beat this deadly foe. But then a routine scan showed a spot in his lung and several in his liver. The lung they could radiate, but not the liver, so Scott began an additional five weeks of radiation and intravenous infusions of chemotherapy, which left him very weak and nauseous. He lost another twenty pounds. Through it all, he worked and fished.

Last summer, I was planning my first fishing trip to Alaska, accompanied by my best friend and my son-in-law. At the last minute, I thought of including Scott. I checked with our host in Alaska and, assured it was no problem to include another fisherman, I asked Scott.

"Have you ever been to Alaska, Scott?"

"No, but I have always wanted to go."

"I'm going in a month with Hurley and Steven. Want to go?"

I will never forget the light in Scott's eyes as he considered the fulfillment of a lifelong dream.

"I'd love to," he said simply and it was done.

Several weeks before we left, Scott began to develop severe headaches. Almost paralyzing, migraine-like, they made even the simplest of tasks nearly impossible. They were explained as a side effect of his chemotherapy. A combination of powerful pain medication and a relatively new migraine medicine made them almost tolerable, but a single dose of the migraine medication was $30 and Scott had no health insurance.

Alaska was beautiful beyond words: blue-green, mirror-like passages dotted with fir-covered islands, whales breaching beside the boat, bald eagles warily watching from the bleached tops of lifeless pines. Scott, the consummate fisherman, was in his element. He and our host, Dave, compared notes on everything from reels to filleting knives. And the first one to land a fish, a beautiful halibut, was Scott. Despite a little nausea, a delayed side effect of the chemo (he never got seasick), Scott had a beautiful twenty-five-pound king salmon, a limit of three halibut, and several snapper within two hours of reaching the fishing grounds. I remember so well the look of happiness and contentment on his face as we motored in through the glassy inland waterways, headed home. Each of the three days we fished was magical for Scott, but he fought mightily against the pounding in his head. And when he had the headaches, he could hardly function. With effort, we arrived home with a beaming Scott and a hundred pounds of frozen halibut and salmon.

The day after we returned, my suspicions were confirmed by an MRI of Scott's brain. It showed two tumors, one golf-ball-sized behind his right eye (the site of the headaches), the other marble-sized in the brain stem at the base of the brain. The first was operable, the second not; however, it could be treated with radiation. That same night, the frontal tumor was removed, and five days after the surgery, Scott began radiation. Miraculously, the headaches disappeared. Soon hairless on his scalp, Scott was guaranteed by the radiation oncologist that he could save his beard, and a form-fitting lead shield was constructed to maintain his facial hair. I shaved my head a bit closer than usual in solidarity with Scott. Instead of having bad hair days, we laughed that we had no hair days.

The radiation and the chemo destroyed the brain tumors, but there was ever-growing concern about the tumors in the liver and around the kidneys. Scott would undergo chemo once a week, a four-hour intravenous infusion of poisons designed to kill the rapidly growing cells of the tumor in preference over the normal cells of his body. Unfortunately, the poisons can't tell the bad cells from the good. Any rapidly growing cells, such as bone marrow, skin, hair, and cells lining the gastrointestinal tract, are susceptible to the chemotherapy. For two days after the chemo, Scott would feel reasonably okay. Then, he would become very ill. The principal side effect was an intractable nausea. "Like the worst seasick you've ever imagined," Scott would explain. Ironically, he'd never been seasick a day in his life. He took pride in the fact that he could fish the roughest seas and never have a problem. But the chemo was different. There were drugs to ease the nausea, but they had their own set of side effects. Some caused extreme drowsiness, some caused involuntary twitching and contraction of muscles, and still others caused headaches.

Through it all, Scott kept working, fishing, and going to Alcoholics Anonymous meetings. He had a number of jobs in progress. He was too weak to work a full day at his normal pace, so several good friends in the building business pitched in and helped him complete them. He bought a fancy "new" used boat with a friend, and together they revamped it and took it on some weekend excursions to the Sacramento River delta for striped bass and for sturgeon.

But Scott was losing his battle against cancer. The repeated scans showed more numerous and larger tumors, and the nausea and weakness were exhausting. Scott quit chemo and tried an alternative herbal treatment, but the herbs made him as sick as the chemo. Fighter that he was, he never stopped looking for an answer. Having beat alcohol and cocaine addiction sixteen years before, he felt he could beat anything.

He had just started yet another chemo when he turned yellow and the pain started in earnest. The liver tumors were obstructing bile ducts, backing the bile up into the circulation and making him jaundiced. And the blockage of the ducts caused pain similar to an attack of gallstones. Biliary colic is known by physicians to be one of the most excruciating pains that patients experience.

With each crescendo of pain, Scott's oncologist responded with a stronger and more effective medication. But the liver blockage also increased the ammonia and other toxins in Scott's blood, causing him to gradually lose his grip on reality. Ironically, although Scott's sixteen years of sobriety meant that he would never die of liver failure from alcohol, he was to die from liver failure caused by his squamous cancer.

With each passing day, Scott became more yellow, gaunter, and a bit more infantile. In bed, he made strange grimacing expressions, and lying on his back, he picked at his bedclothes as if they had small specks of lint on them. He disassembled the fax machine trying "to fix" what wasn't broken, and his wife or one of the family had to watch him constantly as he roamed the house because he would "fix" the computer, the television, his fishing gear, and the coffeemaker.

He stopped eating and drank only small sips when prompted or when medication was required. After what seemed an eternity, he finally went to bed for the last time, while his strong young heart and body fought death for three long days.

Cancer won the corporal battle. Scott won the spiritual battle, however, and the battle over his addiction. When our dear mutual friend, Bud, spoke at his memorial, he announced that Scott had attained a lifetime goal they each had from the beginning, from "the creation" of their sobriety.

He had died sober.

And Scott would not have us mourn his passing. He had lived sixteen years beyond the closet, saved by the love and support of skilled and insightful people. Scott had created a rich new life working, fishing, loving, and sharing his story with anyone who would listen.

It's just that his second life was too short. Scott died two months and twenty-three days short of his forty-fifth birthday.

Bud's Insight

I asked my friend, Bud, why people drink. Lots of reasons, really: grief, sadness, depression, pain, illness, and anger. Grief over the loss of loved ones, of prostates and colons and breasts. Sadness that life is passing us by and so many of our dreams are unreachable. Depression from getting older and more infirm but no closer to the truth. Pain, psychic and physical, and our seeming helplessness to allay or prevent it. Illness that afflicts us without rhyme, reason, or predestination from the universe. And anger. Intense anger. Anger at everything and nothing. Anger at the helplessness and hopelessness of the world. Anger at the greed, evil, injustice, poverty, and misery that have no end.

And no reason.
And no solution.
And so we drink.

15

LARRY, THE SARCASTIC DRUNK

Ever since I was a kid, I wouldn't watch a tragic movie twice. I couldn't accept the ending. When I saw *Dances with Wolves* the second time, I had to turn it off before the soldiers shot Dunbar's wolf and his idyllic world fell apart. Witnessing Larry slip into the depths of an alcoholic's personal hell was similar, except I couldn't change the channel. I had to watch the deterioration of a dear friend as alcohol consumed his life and mind. It was painful to observe because I knew exactly what was happening and why; it was exasperating because I was powerless to help.

Larry has always been a heavy drinker. Beer mostly. After high school, he worked for the gas company for thirty-five years. The workday always ended by downing at least a six-pack with "the boys." Larry used to race motorcycles but twenty years ago began riding a bicycle and running some. Despite his conversion from motor sports to running and cycling, he never changed his persona from the long-haired, bearded biker that he had become in his thirties. Larry was a late-comer to the running craze but became interested in triathlons during their initial popularity. Possessing the hydrodynamic properties of a rock, Larry was nevertheless a decent runner and excelled at the bike. He got heavily into cycling, working up to centuries (100 miles), double centuries (200 miles), and even some ultra-long races requiring several days. Notice the complete, perhaps excessive, immersion in an activity which is so characteristic of the addictive personality. Larry has one.

I met him in 1985 when I was recruited to run the marathon portion of the "World's Toughest Triathlon" at Lake Tahoe. A good running friend had turned triathlete and, as the designated swimmer, organized the team. He would do the 2.4-mile swim in the icy waters of Lake Tahoe, Larry would do the 120-mile bike ride over four high-altitude passes in the surrounding Sierra Nevada, and I would run the 26.2-mile marathon, which climbed to over ten thousand feet.

I was taken aback when I first met Larry. Even then he looked like a derelict. An unkempt gray-white beard framed a flushed face covered with crusty patches from a lifetime of sun damage and drinking. A foul mouth and a blustering demeanor were a bit off-putting, but there was a softer side to Larry: an honest goodness that he couldn't disguise with the rough exterior. We became friends.

Partly due to my example and that of several other friends, Larry took up long-distance running. Although he was considerably slower than I, we would occasionally train together. I had completed the grueling Western States 100-mile run, and I coached Larry in how to train and prepare. He successfully completed it and we planned a trip to Colorado to run the severe, high-altitude Leadville 100-miler. We trained and traveled together with our wives, successfully completed the run, and had a wonderful time.

During this period, Larry would drink heavily and occasionally become rude and obnoxious, but remarkably he was able to discern when he was about to go too far and insult someone. He always stopped short. I was drinking throughout this time, and beer was something we shared, part of the mortar that cemented our relationship. Despite his bluster, rough appearance, and foul mouth, Larry was a genuinely good person, which made it hard to understand why he felt the need to play the role of borderline obnoxious biker dude. Only later, when things really fell apart for him and for our friendship, did I begin to understand. After six months of sobriety and having gained insights into the psychodynamics of alcoholism, I was able to analyze Larry's actions and ascribe meaning to his behavior.

Larry drinks because he is shy and has social anxiety. You'd never believe that if you met him, because he's loud, in-your-face, and very funny when he's drunk. Sober, he is very insecure. Although he is innately very bright, he had little formal education and worked a menial job for thirty-five years. Many of his friends in the running group are college-educated with postgraduate degrees. Larry is aware of the social distance and quite sensitive about it. To compound this, Larry is not comfortable with his appearance. He wears a scraggly biker beard to disguise his physical defects. Alcohol and attitude hide his social shortcomings.

It is a basic human need to feel liked and wanted. Over time, people develop strategies to achieve those goals and to compensate for detrimental personality and/or physical traits. When Larry drank, he became exceedingly funny. He was very perceptive at determining others' weaknesses and exploiting them. If someone was fat, bald, short, old, whatever, Larry seized that defect, made fun of it, and immediately had that person on the defensive. A person who is flawed and hypersensitive develops the ability to find the flaws in others and exploit them. Larry was very good at it, dominating almost any social gathering and reaffirming that the best defense is a good offense. He was masterful at ridicule, taking his remarks to the edge of cruelty but not beyond. He would keep his social adversaries slightly off-balance, which he felt would keep them from looking at his shortcomings and attacking them. The cost of being Larry's friend was having a thick skin and being able to laugh about your flaws because he invariably found them and highlighted them for you and everyone else in the room.

In the last several years, Larry's body began to show the signs of years of intense physical work. Knee problems curtailed his running and began to affect his cycling. The natural antidepressant effect of the exercise was gone, and Larry began to drink more, trying to make himself feel better. The beer gave way to "toddies," first in the evening on the weekends and then every evening. Toddies were hard liquor, with or without mix. The toddy of choice was Canadian whiskey and Seven-Up: three or four ounces of whiskey in a tall tumbler full of ice, topped off with Seven-Up.

During the summer of 2001, Larry and his wife agreed to drive and crew for my wife and me on an eight-week cross-country horse ride. From the outset, I knew something was wrong. Larry would begin drinking beer at 9 or 10 AM, and he switched to the toddy tumbler by two or three in the afternoon. The ride and the crewing were very hard work, with long hours in the heat and constant attention to equipment problems, horse needs, and logistical details. Rising at 3:30 AM every morning, we had to be prepared to be on the horse and on the road at 5 AM to beat the sweltering Midwestern summer heat. Dinner, preparations for the next day, and the late sunset kept us from getting to sleep until 10 or 11 PM. It was grueling for me, and I was sober and in good physical shape.

Alcohol doesn't permit restful sleep. It alters a particularly vital kind of sleep associated with dreaming called rapid eye movement (REM) sleep. With few hours to sleep and the quality of his rest impaired, Larry began to unravel. He started to forget things and make mistakes suggesting his attention was impaired. He drove the truck away from the trailer with the auxiliary power cord still hooked up, ripping the plug out of its receptacle. One morning after a particularly heavy night with the toddies and frequent coal trains going by the fairgrounds where we were camped, Larry filled the motor home gas tank with water. His normal helpful nature was replaced with a grudging obedience. He never smiled. Half-gallon after half-gallon of whiskey disappeared. One afternoon and evening I counted five toddies, after six or eight beers. That represents between sixteen and thirty ounces of alcohol. Scabs and large bruises began to appear on Larry's shins from falling down. Drunk in the wee hours, he would stagger back to the trailer from benders with some of the other crews. His mood degenerated from gray to black and he responded in monosyllables. His vulgar language and humor became vile and hurtful. Totally miserable and unable to understand why, Larry relied even more on his old friend, alcohol, to make him feel better and lift his spirits. The more he drank, the worse he felt and acted.

The hard work, heat, lack of sleep, and alcohol were too much for Larry. If the trip had lasted another month, he may well have had an alcoholic-psychotic break. As it was, he was dangerously close. I sent him home a week early, unable to deal with his ugliness and the pain I felt at watching a dear friend destroy himself.

Larry came home and almost immediately told everyone he knew that he was moving. He didn't like living in this area anymore; he needed a change. In the AA vernacular, such a move is called a "geographic." The alcoholic is miserable but in denial as to the cause. He searches for a reason other than the obvious, and all the little annoyances about his living circumstance become magnified. He decides that his unhappiness must be the result of where he lives, so he moves. And he takes the misery and the alcohol with him. He is just as unhappy and in just as much denial, but now he's in a different place. Alcoholics can run but they can't hide. Their problem is always with them.

I've seen Larry at a couple of parties since we got back from our ride. I worked hard at forgiving him, since his behavior had come close to ruining a trip my wife and I had been planning for several years and in which we had heavily invested financially and physically. But I have learned the importance of forgiveness to my spiritual and emotional health and I was successful. The first time I saw him was a very awkward moment. I stuck out my hand and said hello. He refused my gesture, turned away, and grumbled something under his breath. I understand. I remind him of a sad part of his life that he is unwilling to examine or to change. I won't accept responsibility for his unhappiness. And I know from my understanding of alcoholism and my own experience that his problem has complete control of him. And no matter where he goes or what he does, it will not go away. He's not the same Larry that I met eighteen years ago and learned to love. There is no twinkle in his eye, no joy in his voice. Behind the jokes and the insulting sarcasm, there no longer exists humor. There is anger, bitterness, and confusion. Larry can feel that something is very wrong. He is miserable but doesn't know why. He blames the infirmities of his age, the place he lives, the relationships with his kids, or the friends who have abandoned him. All the while, the noose of alcohol tightens its grip and further distorts the truth. Perilously close to a free fall into oblivion, Larry has distanced himself from the few friends that might be able to help when the crisis comes.

And sooner or later, it will.

Dateline: TEXAS

MAN GETS LIFE FOR KILLING
FRIEND OVER LAST BEER

A jury gave a life sentence to a Bandera man who shot and killed a longtime friend he accused of drinking the last beer in his refrigerator. Jurors deliberated less than two hours before passing the sentence on Steven Brasher, 42, for the Nov. 5, 2001, murder of Willie Lawson, 39.
"There was only two beers left, so I took one, and I told Willie not to take my last beer," Brasher said in a taped statement that was played for jurors during the trial. San Luis Obispo Telegram Tribune.

Do you think Steve was sober at the time?

16

MARC, THE MEAN DRUNK

o o o o o o o o o o o o o o o o o o o o o o o o o o o o o o o o o o o

"Instant Asshole: just add alcohol"

—baseball cap logo

For every drunk who is seemingly humorous like Larry, there's one who is mean and angry. It took me years to realize how angry alcohol made me. Just one beer would change my personality and make me more argumentative. I had seen my dad get surly and quarrelsome at the dinner table when he drank, and there were guys in the fraternity house who got drunk and put their fists through walls. But I had never seen a really mean drunk up close until I met Marcus Barr.

Marc Barr was in my internship class at Los Angeles County-USC Medical Center. He was a straight surgery intern, headed for a residency in the Ear, Nose, and Throat field (ENT). Marc was six feet two, 220 pounds, and every pound was rock-hard muscle. He had been an all-American linebacker at a big southeastern university. Ruggedly handsome with a chiseled jaw and thick black hair, he was smart, friendly, and a genuinely nice guy. That is, when he was sober.

Thursday night was "boys' night out" during our internship. Anybody who didn't have duty or wasn't too exhausted from the previous night's call gathered after dinner in the staff cafeteria, piled into cars, and swarmed to one of the local watering holes, either in Santa Monica or Pasadena. I was married and had already done the bar scene in college, but occasionally I'd tag along.

One night in late summer, several months into the internship, I joined the group at the Oar House in Santa Monica. My constant companion and partner on many rotations, Joe Fertig, went along, as did a dozen or so of my fellow interns. Marc Barr was among them.

Clustered in a small knot, drinking beer and eating popcorn, we occupied one end of the long bar, checking out the women and swapping lies about college and med school exploits. After a half hour and a couple of beers, Fertig turned to me.

"Barr's got that look in his eyes." Joe had gone to med school with the linebacker.

I shrugged my shoulders with a questioning look.

"He's looking for a fight."

I regarded Barr. He was not laughing and talking with the rest. He was preoccupied, looking over their shoulders, surveying the crowd at the bar. There was a set to his jaw and fierceness in his eyes that I had never seen. After several minutes, he left the group and wandered down the bar.

"Watch this," Fertig said.

Three-quarters of the way down the room, Barr hesitated and then approached the bar. He bumped shoulders with a large and particularly boisterous man. The man turned, glared at Marc, and said something. Marc's back was toward us but I saw him shake a finger at the bigger man, who suddenly tensed, drew himself up to his full height, straightened his shoulders, and stared at Barr, who gestured toward the door.

"There he goes. That bozo doesn't know what he's in for."

"I don't get it," I said, confused.

"Marc loves to fight. After a few beers, he picks out the toughest guy at the bar and picks a fight with him."

"You're serious?"

"You always want to look wimpy when Marc's had a few." We watched the two men exit the bar. Ten minutes later, Barr reentered alone and swaggered over to the bar. The pocket of his shirt was nearly torn off; his right ear was swollen. The knuckles of both hands were scraped and bleeding.

"I showed that asshole," he said, and picked up his beer.

Marc was a prime example of a type of alcoholic who has a drastic and negative personality change when he's drunk. Sober, he was pleasant, courteous, very respectful of women, and smart enough to get through medical school with above-average grades. But deep inside was anger, a violence, a need to dominate and feel powerful—all unleashed with alcohol. Alcohol is a solvent both chemically and psychologically. It removes inhibitions and social restraint. This is the type of drunk who might abuse his wife or his kids. Alcohol is, for people like Marc, the excuse for losing control. And sadly, society too often condones it. When we hear that Phil Brown struck his wife, the comment, "He was drinking," somehow explains it or makes it acceptable. There are, in many social circles, two sets of behavioral standards: one for the sober person and one for the drunk, as if being drunk somehow makes violent or antisocial actions okay. It is this double standard, this willingness of large segments of our culture to tolerate the violence created by intoxication, that abets much of the child abuse and spousal abuse that is epidemic in our nation.

There's more to the tale of Marc Barr. He had a couple of dozen fights that internship year. Then one spring morning, after a long Friday night on call, I saw Joe Fertig in the cafeteria. He walked over and sat down beside me.

"Did you hear about Barr?"

"No, what happened?"

"He was at the Oar House last night with some of the guys. He hadn't been there ten minutes when some guy tapped him on the shoulder. Marc turned and this guy hit him in the eye with the broken end of a beer bottle."

The imagery was sickening. I could see the jagged end of the bottle twisting into the orbit.

"Did he lose the eye?"

"Not sure yet. He's still in surgery. Some people say he finally got what was coming to him."

Despite the best medical care possible, Marc did lose his eye, and a month of his internship. After three surgeries, the cheek and lid scars were repaired in an acceptable manner. I saw him from a distance in the hallway but I didn't encounter him personally. I didn't want to, as I wouldn't know what to say. I viewed it as a terrible tragedy, but, like Fertig, I felt that Marc had brought it on himself. Or rather, the person that Marc became when he drank had attracted an even more violent and vengeful drunk, one who didn't play by the same set of rules, one who lost even more control when he was intoxicated. Alcohol and the violent personalities it creates account for 50 percent of the homicides in this country each year (Student Affairs Handbook 2005–2006).

I lost track of Marc after that year. I heard he went on to pursue the ENT career. Hopefully, his life-altering loss generated some introspective reflection and Marc realized that alcohol was a factor. The simple two-carbon fragment that impairs judgment had altered his life forever.

17

REX ALAN KREBS: ALCOHOL CREATES SOME MONSTERS

He kidnapped two beautiful young women, raped them multiple times, strangled both, and buried them in shallow graves.

My picturesque, friendly town had been wracked with the most gut-wrenching terror imaginable. In a place where few people used to lock their front doors, and anyone was safe walking the streets at night, two beautiful young college girls were violently murdered and buried in shallow graves only a few miles from the breathtaking canyon that I call home. The entire community felt violated and still has not recovered. The image remains of helicopters overhead searching for graves and FBI agents strolling up my driveway and into the orchard to flash their credentials and begin asking questions.

In the end, they arrested a short, balding man in his mid-thirties with a prior conviction for rape, and as the story unfolded, alcohol was as much the murder weapon as the rope he wound around the two coeds' necks.

Rex Alan Krebs became very evil when he drank.

He survived an abusive childhood, and in the early 1990s, he found his way to the central coast of California. One night, after he was rebuffed by a young woman whose look of disdain touched a nerve in his intoxicated and self-conscious brain, he followed her home, waited until she was asleep, broke into her apartment, hog-tied her, and raped her. In his alcohol-fogged brain, he had gotten even. But he got caught and went to prison.

Four years later, he was released and returned to the Central Coast. He rented a house in a rural area from a lady he met at church. He told her that he had been in prison for rape but that it was a bum rap. He described a "date rape" of a woman who willingly had sex with him and then had remorse. The story was nothing like the court records of his brutal assault. But the landlady took pity on the young man and rented to him, never checking his story or sharing his past with her neighbors.

He took a job at a local lumberyard as a salesclerk. Even sober, there was evidence of his intent. He kept a list of the phone numbers and addresses of all the pretty female customers he waited on. It was simple to copy that vital and sensitive information from the checks they wrote for their purchases.

A condition of his parole was that he could not drink alcohol. It was recognized, and Krebs acknowledged that he became psychotic when he drank. He accepted the terms of his release. But he began taking home a six-pack of beer after work. He even bought some for a next-door neighbor's live-in girlfriend and flirted with her on his drive up the canyon.

Then one night, after drinking, he followed a young woman on her way home from a restaurant in town. By all accounts, she'd had too much to drink and had a long walk. As she crossed a large steel bridge over the railroad tracks, he attacked, knocking her senseless. Then he carried her to his truck and drove her to his remote house, far enough from neighbors that no one could observe his actions or hear her screams. The terror she endured during her last hours is unthinkable.

A month later, he struck again. This time, he crawled through a young woman's bathroom window and beat, bound, and kidnapped her. Back in the canyon, the macabre scenario played out again, and he buried his second victim close beside the first.

Krebs's parole officer's astute observations put an end to the murders. He noticed a toy gun and beer cans in Rex's house, violations of his parole. He also observed a limp and some bruises that couldn't have come from "cutting wood," as the parolee alleged.

Rex Krebs is in prison, by his own admission a "monster" that should be eliminated. But sober, he worked, dated, went to church, and carried on a seemingly normal life. Once he drank, he transformed into a sinister brute beyond our comprehension.

So why would he ever drink? Surely, he understood that alcohol transformed him into a monster. Certainly, in sober reflection, he would never want to perform those inhuman acts on innocent human beings. He would never want to go back to prison. So why would he drink again?

Because, alcohol made Rex feel good and he liked the feeling. When he drank he felt better about himself—no longer short, fat, bald, and unattractive to women. He felt handsome and irresistibly sexually attractive. He knew he had a problem with alcohol and that knowledge would keep him out of trouble: he'd be on guard. But alcohol is seductive. After the first few "feel-good" beers, the next few depressed him. He really was short and fat and bald and most women wouldn't look at him twice. And the next few beers made him angry. God help the woman who gave Rex Alan Krebs a look of disdain after that sixth beer. His rage, resulting from feelings of inadequacy developed during an abusive childhood and reinforced by his lonely life, rose up in him, and neither insight into his alcohol-induced behavior nor the fear of prison could stop it. Besides, his alcohol-deluded mind reasoned, last time he got caught because she accused him. This time there would be no survivor. He reasoned that the rape and murder were the violence he owed a world that despised him. He was just getting even, and the alcohol flowing in his veins made it happen, released him from any restraint a sober mind would feel. It turned Rex Krebs into an animal so devoid of feeling that he could choke the life from the bodies of his victims.

Society will now have its pound of flesh. And by a rationale no less misguided than Krebs's, it will torture him with years on death row, last-minute appeals, and preparations for a lethal injection. Maybe it will eliminate him, or maybe it will warehouse him for life, but the years of uncertainty and fear will be a "cruel and unusual punishment" for a man who can't really understand what happened to him or why. All he knows is that alcohol makes him crazy, yet he allowed it to take over and destroy his life.

Society makes rules and has sanctions for breaking those rules. They are based on our Judeo-Christian heritage and on the understandable need for individuals and groups who live in close proximity to act civilly toward one another, avoiding mayhem and anarchy. Alcohol often blinds people to society's rules. I listened to an interview with a Serbian soldier accused of the mass murder of Muslim women and children in Croatia. He explained that he had been drinking when the order came to gun down the prisoners. That made it easier, he said. Besides, if he didn't carry out the order, he feared he would be shot as well. Fortunately, we don't have a set of rules for sober behavior and another for drunkenness. Yet, too often we accept that there are. "Oh, he was just drunk," we alibi for someone's appalling actions. Is there a difference between the husband who verbally abuses his wife, the Serbian soldier, and Rex Krebs?

Only in degree. If a person has dark tendencies when he or she drinks, constraint has been lost. There's no telling how far the behavior will escalate once the reasoning mind is stupefied.

"Have a beer.
Give your brain the night off."

—Logo on a baseball cap

18

I HAVE AN EXCUSE

He sat trembling, pulling little scabs off the back of his hand. He would hold them up to me as proof of the worms he had seen crawling out of his skin.

"See. Here's one of them. Now you'll believe me."

Ronnie had delusions of parasitosis, believing that he had critters burrowing out of his skin. It is a disease characteristically caused by specific drug abuse.

"Is it coke or meth, Ronnie?"

"It's crank, Doc. And booze."

"Aren't you tired of being a slave to it? It owns you."

"Yeah, Doc, I am. Maybe sometime I'll quit, but not right now. There's too much stress. I can't get over losing my dad."

"There's always gonna be something, Ronnie."

"Doc, you'd drink and do crank too if you'd been through what I've been through."

One of the common story threads of the majority of alcoholics is that they drink for good reason and it is almost never their fault. In medical school and throughout my medical career, I've noticed that alcoholics as a group can always justify their behavior. With apologies to my psychologist/psychiatrist colleagues, I divide much of the world's psychopathology into two personality types: neurosis and character disorder. Neurotics blame themselves for everything. If grandma fell and broke her hip at the nursing home, it was because the neurotic person forgot to call her that day. You get the idea. Those with a character disorder are just the opposite: It's never their fault. If they run a red light and broadside someone in an intersection, it's because the sun blinded them through the windshield and they couldn't see the signal. So they sue the city for placing the signal improperly. Alcohol abusers fit in the latter category, as a rule. Their drinking and the behavior that it produces is not their fault.

Harold was a career alcoholic. I admitted him twice during my stint on the overdose ward at LA County-USC Medical Center. As he sobered up, he always would get weepy and blubber about how it was "all her fault." "Her" was his wife, Sarah, who left him after five years of marriage because she couldn't live with his drinking. He'd been through three jobs, had been in the detox unit five times, and had two DUIs. Sarah went through counseling, joined Al-Anon, and got Harold into an alcohol rehab program but eventually felt Harold didn't want to quit, so she opted out of their marriage. It is a startling revelation for the loved one to discover that the alcoholic chooses alcohol over his mate. But given the nature of addiction, it is true. The sooner the alcoholic's spouse comes to that realization and separates herself, the better. By staying with the alcoholic, praying that he will recover, she is enabling him to continue drinking. By leaving him, she is appropriately attaching negative consequences to the addiction. Sarah prayed that the initial separation and the possible conditional return would be the motivation Harold needed to quit. It was not. It simply provided him with a reason to continue drinking. Whatever previous excuse Harold used before his separation, forever after it was the cruelty of his wife leaving him that created his grief. And it really was unquenchable: first with vodka and whiskey, and later when he really hit the skids, it was with cheap port and Tokay. The divorce made drinking so much easier for Harold, as he rationalized that it was his wife's fault. His grief was so overwhelming that it was uncontrollable. He had to drink. Notice how subtly Harold had changed the argument. His drinking was not the problem. It was the grief, and Sarah was to blame.

Joe was an alcoholic I treated during my residency at the Veterans Administration Hospital in Long Beach. He had terrible psoriasis. 50 percent of his body was covered with huge red scaly patches. For the uninitiated, the appearance of severe psoriasis is grotesque. These patients have a terrible social stigma, and many of them drink to try to cope with their feelings of denigration. As I explained previously, the irony is that heavy drinking exacerbates psoriasis. So the binges and the flares of psoriasis go hand in hand. In fact, scientific papers have looked at whether alcoholism might trigger the onset or flaring of psoriasis in susceptible individuals.

Joe would come in after two weeks of hard drinking. His psoriasis would be out of control and oftentimes secondarily infected with strep or staph bacteria. I would dry him out, treat the infection, put him in our ultraviolet light cabinet, get his psoriasis well on the way to clearing up, and then send him out to repeat the cycle all over again.

"You don't know what it's like, Doc. My life is hell. You should try to live with this crap." And he was right, I didn't know. Thirty years later, I have taken care of hundreds of patients with psoriasis and I know it is one of life's great challenges. But, I take care of some very high-profile state and local officials, a very successful attorney, several physicians, and many other highly successful people with psoriasis who don't need to use it as an excuse to drink. They meet the challenge and, in conquering it, make the other challenges in their lives more attainable.

Alcoholics will use any excuse as a justification for their problem. One of the worst drunks I treated at LA County-USC was a mid-thirties woman whose life spun out of control after she lost a baby to a third-trimester miscarriage in her mid-twenties. She drank heavily during the pregnancy, and her grief at the loss may have been mixed with a large dose of subconscious guilt at perhaps contributing to the stillbirth. It may have been a blessing that she did lose the baby. If she had carried it to term, the child quite possibly would have had fetal alcohol syndrome, which is a devastating side effect of maternal alcohol consumption.

There are untold numbers of alcoholics who were unloved or abused as children, who are drunk because they hate work or lost their job. Perhaps they flunked out of medical school, lost the big promotion, or their mom/dad/spouse/brother/sister/twin died of cancer. Any negative circumstance is an excuse to drink. They so brilliantly change the focus from their drinking to some life-altering event that "caused" them to drink. Then, they are not to blame.

Most alcohol abusers believe that drinking helps them to cope with their difficult lives. Alcohol doesn't help anyone cope with anything. At the end of the first or second drink, there is a "feel-good" moment that produces a nanosecond of bliss, but it is followed by stupor and, in time, by depression. Add depression to whatever it is that originally created the need to drink and the problem only gets worse.

So what does the problem drinker do?

Drink some more.

But it never works. It just widens the chasm and deepens the abyss of despair until, in time, they are free-falling headlong into it.

19

ALCOHOL WILL MAKE YOU CRAZY: THE NATIVE AMERICAN EXPERIENCE

o o o o o o o o o o o o o o o o o o o o o o o o o o o o o o o o o o o

"Brothers: Why would you drink the fire-water, and become fools? Would it not be better that the Long-knife no more bring it to us? We give for it our robes and our horse—it does us no good. It makes us poor. We fight our own brothers and kill those we love, because the fire-water is in us and makes our hearts bad! The fire-water is the red man's enemy."

—*Bull Tail, Lakota chief, 1841, two days before he tried to trade his daughter, Chintzille, for a keg of whiskey. (Nadeau)*

Among the great tragedies of human history is the demise of the Native American peoples, crushed beneath the avalanche of Western European culture as it expanded into the New World. No more effective dismantling and eroding of these societies could have been accomplished with premeditation, than occurred in the eighteenth- and nineteenth-centuries in what was becoming the United States. If it had been a planned military campaign, it could not have been as devastating as were the naturally occurring events when a Stone Age culture interfaced with the embryonic industrialized world.

Willfully or not, Western European explorers and colonists waged biological and chemical warfare against Native Americans. Late in the eighteenth century, measles decimated the populations of Native peoples living in contact with settlers on the eastern seaboard. As the newly designated "Americans" moved westward, they brought alien infectious diseases for which the indigenous people had no natural immunity. There is an incredible account of a tainted blanket carried up the Missouri River on a steamboat. Wherever that boat docked, a plague of smallpox exploded into the surrounding countryside. Europeans, whose ancestors had been exposed to the highly contagious and virulent disease, lost 30 percent of those infected with the grotesque draining blisters that covered the entire body. But for the hapless Native Americans, whose immune systems had never encountered this member of the *Herpes humanis* family, the mortality was nearly 90 percent. Whole villages were devastated. A better biological warfare agent does not exist.

Then began the chemical warfare. Kegs of alcohol traveled up the rivers in bullboats and steamboats and across the prairie in wagons and on mules. And again, the traders and early trappers could not have picked a better agent. It killed many but also eroded the social fabric of the culture and enslaved an entire people.

Exploration and settling of the West began with Lewis and Clark in 1804. Not far behind were explorers and trappers, responding to the European world's desire for furs, who found it expeditious to buy or trade with the Indian tribes. As economic pressure grew, many of the fur companies hired their own trappers.

Because the beaver trade was so lucrative, intense competition developed, principally between the British Hudson Bay Company and the American Fur Company owned by John Jacob Astor. It was British rum versus American whiskey. The traders had learned very early on that they had to have liquor to compete for the Indian furs. In 1830, Peter Skene Ogden employed a group of Rockway Indians to trap for him, but they deserted when Thomas Fitzpatrick offered to trade whiskey for their pelts.

The American government banned trade in liquor with the Native Americans but left a loophole. A gill (four ounces) per day was allowed each man in the trading party. This allowed enormous quantities of alcohol to be shipped up the rivers and carried across the plains.

Congress then moved for a total ban on liquor in the territory. Astor complained to a member of Congress that, without liquor, competition against the Hudson Bay Company "was hopeless, for the attraction (to the Indians) is irresistible."

And so it was. Without any cultural point of reference or social or religious taboos against it, the Native Americans were overwhelmed. They drank it, they enjoyed it, they became addicted to it, and it created unthinkable consequences.

The stories are incredible. Mothers traded children for a keg of whiskey. Fathers gave marriage-age daughters to the traders but required that a party be held at which the trader was expected to provide the libation. A whole season's work would be traded for liquor. Whiskey was preferred over blankets, iron kettles, ax blades, and knives.

The standard rate of exchange was three cupfuls of liquor for a buffalo hide. Native Americans would claim their due and drink it. They offered it to their wives and children, and when it ran short, they passed it around from mouth to mouth, a single mouthful being passed to as many as twelve friends. And when it was spent, those who drank it would breathe on those who had none, giving them the perfume of the elixir. As the transactions proceeded, the sober trader would cheat the intoxicated Indian. The liquor was diluted with water and, by the end of the trading, the drunken Indian might be drinking plain water.

At times, the bargaining grew violent. Traders were beaten or shot, and the Native Americans often quarreled among themselves. There were stabbings and shootings in the fury of drunkenness. Jesuit missionary Father de Smet recorded thirteen deaths in a three-week period on the Upper Missouri, all involving alcohol.

It was one of the most evil and insidious chapters in Western history: a dignified, proud, and self-reliant people reduced to beggars, whores, and thieves by alcohol. Tribes closer to civilization used their government annuities to buy liquor. By the time the annuity arrived each year, it was already owed on account to the traders.

Liquor inflamed them. They got drunk and fought, not just their enemies but within themselves.

Liquor destroyed them. As one observer recorded:

"They were gay and lighthearted, but they are now moody and melancholy; they were confiding, they are now jealous and sullen; they were athletic and active, they are now impotent and inert; they were just though implacable, they are now malignant and vindictive; they were honorable and dignified, they are now mean and abased; integrity and fidelity were their characteristics, now they are both dishonest and unfaithful; they were brave and courteous, they are now cowardly and abusive. They are melting away before the curse of the white man's friendship…" (Nadeau)

Loved ones of alcoholics often report personality and character changes strikingly similar to those documented in this 150-year-old transcript. In the instance of the Native American, the changes are so obvious and dramatic that they provide an excellent case study of the personal and social degradation produced by liquor in our contemporary culture.

Not all Native Americans succumbed to the seduction of alcohol. Some tribes, with incredible wisdom and restraint, forbade their members to partake. The Pawnee were one such tribe. Asked why the Pawnee didn't drink, one chief sagely observed, "We're crazy enough without it." Pawnee warriors, adorned in tribal finery and mounted on sleek ponies, were a stark contrast to the disheveled tribes stricken with the passion for drink. When alcohol was first introduced on the Plains, some prominent Crow chiefs became very drunk and embarrassed themselves. Later sober and contrite, they banned liquor from their tribe. They called it "fool's water" and poured it on the ground whenever it was found near their encampment.

The great Lakota warrior Crazy Horse would not touch alcohol. With a rich vision of life, he had prescience of the demise of his people and knew that alcohol would play a role in degrading and enslaving them. He led his people in battle soberly and shrewdly, clinging to the hope that he might rally enough followers to save the Lakota way of life and resist the tide of change. Unfortunately, few of his peers shared his vision or heeded his counsel.

When I read of such tragedy as the destruction of an entire culture, abetted by alcohol, I am amazed that its dangerous potential isn't more apparent. It is then that I remember how seductive, how blinding, how addictive alcohol is. Many reading this account would mourn the poor alcoholic Native Americans, who were genetically and culturally unable to handle liquor, while ignoring their two double scotches accompanying dinner and the subsequent fight with a family member.

Certainly, there are social drinkers, people who have a glass of wine once or twice a week with dinner and occasionally at a party. But new studies estimate that 30 percent of Americans who drink alcohol are binge drinkers (Miller 2004). Add to that the percentage of people who "every now and then" have too much to drink and do something foolish that they wouldn't do sober. Many, like myself, are high-functioning alcoholics, but given the right stresses, they can become common drunks. In the case of our Native Americans, history shows that alcohol was integral in the demise of their culture.

Culture and Alcohol

Over dinner the other night, two friends, recovering alcoholics, and I were discussing the different responses various cultures have had to alcohol. My friend Bud (the alcoholic professor) had just returned from Holland, where his wife still has relatives. They go every summer for a few weeks. Bud was marveling at the liberal attitude of the Dutch regarding both alcohol and drugs. They are available and not nearly as tightly controlled as they are in the United States, and yet the Dutch do not seem to have as much trouble with alcoholism and drug abuse as we in America do. Similarly, in France, wine is freely available and drunk by children with meals from a very early age, and yet the culture does not seem to have the problems with it that we Americans do. Scott pointed out that there appears to be a relationship with the length of time that a culture has been exposed to alcohol and the amount of alcoholism. For example, the Jews have had alcohol in their culture for five thousand years, and they don't have nearly the problem with alcohol abuse as Native American cultures with the introduction of alcohol to their societies in the eighteenth and nineteenth centuries.

Bud speculated that there might be some natural selection at work. When alcohol is first introduced to a culture, the most addiction-prone may develop a severe acute addiction and be incapacitated or die from it, removing a portion of the genetically susceptible addictive persons from the gene pool. Thus, the longer a culture has been exposed to alcohol, the fewer alcoholics. Bud related accounts of people who were hopelessly addicted from their first drink and died of alcoholism in short order.

If that were the case, however, you would expect to see decreasing rates of alcoholism in cultures where it was introduced within the last six or eight generations, such as the Native American populations. Most observers would agree that the alcohol abuse problem in these cultures has not diminished in the last fifty years. Some would argue that the introduction of alcohol is still too recent to see the diminution. Also, some would argue that artificially imposed social welfare systems and health care have kept the severe alcoholics from dying out before they have the opportunity to reproduce. It is an interesting idea to ponder.

20

SEE RICK DRINK AND UNDERSTAND WHY

He bent to the task and pulled the skiff in on the long rope. His movements were quick, his strength astonishing. The bottom scraped on the rocky shore as the boat grounded. At seventy-four, Rick move like a man half his age. He had been a lumberjack and roustabout in Alaska for thirty years and an alcoholic for fifty. Five decades of drinking and fighting left little of Rick's dentition.

A buddy of mine hired him to help build a dock. The night before, Rick had beached his boat at 3:00 AM, staggered out, fell on the rocks, and then crawled home. Amazingly, he was there at 7:00 AM to start work, showing no apparent sign of the previous night's debauch. How can he drink that hard and still function the next day?

There are several good explanations. The first and most logical is that he doesn't function nearly as well as he would if he had not been plastered the night before. Rick's liver could not have metabolized all the alcohol he'd consumed the previous night by the time he arrived at work. He still has a significant blood alcohol at 7:00 AM. So how does he function? Simply put, Rick functions at a reasonably effective level still drunk, with a blood alcohol of 0.1 to 0.2 percent. It is a learned skill, like driving drunk. Many people can drive well enough not to be spotted by the highway patrol with a blood alcohol in that range. On tests of subtle motor skills or reaction times, results are abnormal; nevertheless, many function well enough to get by. And of course, as the blood alcohol level drops and symptoms of withdrawal arise, Rick starts drinking again. The amazing fact, for many people like Rick, is that they are virtually never sober. Ever.

How can he maintain a high level of alcohol intake for fifty years and not have cirrhosis? There are many reasons. It may depend on what he drinks. Beer is relatively "liver-friendly" because it doesn't contain a lot of impurities. Distilled spirits are a lot more toxic to the liver. Distillation is the process of boiling a liquid that has been fermented to produce alcohol. The alcohol has a lower boiling point, so it boils before water and is concentrated. However, in the distillation process, many other volatile chemicals such as benzene and toluene are concentrated as well. Many are more toxic to the liver than alcohol. As a result, drinking distilled spirits may render the drunk more likely to develop cirrhosis.

Rick avoided or postponed liver disease by eating well when he drank. Liver cells have an amazing ability to regenerate, but they require a significant amount of protein and vitamins in the diet. If absent, the same amount of alcohol causes more damage because the liver doesn't repair itself as well. Alcoholics may not eat much because they are too drunk to care, or the alcoholic calories satisfy their hunger. When alcohol intake creates a nutritional deficiency, the process of cirrhosis is accelerated.

Finally, there appears to be genetic susceptibility to cirrhosis. Two people can drink the same type and amount of alcohol and have the same diet. One develops cirrhosis and the other doesn't. One liver simply doesn't repair as well as the other after injury from alcohol. Or perhaps more scar tissue is made. It's similar to emphysema and smoking. Some people develop the devastating lung disease with light smoking, while others, like my uncle, can smoke two packs a day for sixty years and not even be short of breath.

The situation with alcohol is not understood as well, but it must have a similar mechanism. Some people repair their alcoholic hepatitis more efficiently, with less scar tissue, than others. Rick, the lumberjack, obviously does. It appears that Rick has a genetically acquired resistance to alcoholic liver disease.

But there's a lot more to Rick than a toothless, drunk lumberman. He has a remarkable intellect. Sometime between work and the nightly intoxication, Rick read voraciously. He checked books out at the library and devoured them. He could discuss any of the great classics in depth. Considering he was drunk most of the time, how did he read, digest, and remember all those books? Rick may represent the 1 percent of the population that can drink excessively and function both physically and intellectually at a very high level. Again, it may be attributed to incredible genes.

Yet what a loss to society! Rick could have been an inspiring teacher or writer. To see an intellect such as his wasted on drunken discussions of *Hamlet* is a shame.

Curiosity about Rick's life choices is heightened by the knowledge that he has two brothers, both of whom are very accomplished. One is a prominent physician in the Boston area, the other a CEO of a NASDAQ company. It's clear that Rick didn't get all the brains, but he got his share. Why did he choose to squander this gift? Rick was the youngest of three brothers. It is a common scenario in the dynamics of family life that second and third siblings, feeling that they cannot successfully compete with an older and very accomplished sibling, choose alternate goals, lifestyles, and pathways. That is certainly the case with Rick. Under the guise of his alcoholism, he simply refused to compete with his older brothers.

Alcohol often serves a psychological need in the beginning. Once the addiction is well-established, it maintains a life of its own.

Many alcoholics drink to ease psychic pain resulting from lack of parental love, lack of self-esteem, death of a loved one, or a broken marriage. The long list of precipitating factors can also include estranged parents or children, physical pain and disability, shyness, disappointment at not fulfilling a life goal, or, for the overly empathetic, the inability to cope with the great pain and sorrow in our society.

The world has always been replete with pain and suffering. There has always been injustice, poverty, illness, hatred, and evil. It is not a question of whether or not we will experience pain, but how we deal with it.

In America, we live in a "fix it" culture. It is often thought that our modern technological world has the solution to any problem. If we can reprogram a satellite a hundred miles into space, we should be able to solve our problems here on earth. We expect solutions, and being the impatient people that we are, we want the solution right now. We are also a "feel-good" society. Great social significance is placed on being happy, being fulfilled, and finding meaning in life.

So, in summary, we want and expect happiness right now. We want to understand why we are not happy, and we want and expect to fix it right now.

And when these expectations are not met, what do we do? We change jobs. We get a divorce. We get angry. We drink or take drugs. We escape from the problem. We are not willing to endure the stress, pain, or conflict, and let it temper us. We are not willing to accept that there is no immediate answer and that we simply have to "be" with the problem awhile to let it transform us into stronger, humbler, more serene people. We are not willing to be humbled by the problem. We are not willing to ask for help outside of ourselves.

And so we have higher-than-ever rates of divorce, suicide, alcoholism and drug abuse, violent crime, spousal and child abuse, dissatisfaction, and medical illness.

Sadly, alcohol never solves the problem. It just eases the pain for a time. When we sober up, it remains unsolved. As a friend in recovery put it, "Your life can never be so messed up that alcohol can't make it worse."

NEVER SOBER

If you drink every day, you are never completely sober, completely without the effect of alcohol in your system. There are spaces within the body where fluids exist, the constituents of which are altered very slowly. The aqueous humor in the front or anterior chamber of the eye and the vitreous humor behind the lens are two such spaces. Alcohol is removed very slowly from these areas, so slowly, in fact, that forensic pathologists can measure the alcohol level in these fluids postmortem and determine, with great accuracy, the blood alcohol level and the state of sobriety or inebriation of the deceased for several days before death. Alcohol also persists in isolated areas of the brain and in alterations to the chemical messengers in nerve cells. So, for many who drink every day, they are always under the influence.

21

BUD, THE ALCOHOLIC COLLEGE PROFESSOR

He looked and acted the part: tan and athletic, with a keen mind and a friendly handshake. A triathlete who also completed double-century bike races, he was a noted professor of history at our local university. And no matter what time of the day, he always smelled of liquor. I marveled at how he could do it, and I noted that he was increasingly inebriated each time I saw him in the office. Then, suddenly, he disappeared. He had serious skin cancer problems and I saw him regularly every three months, so when his appointments stopped, I figured he must have changed doctors. Or, maybe he died of alcoholism.

Almost.

When Bud Beecher returned for a visit, the tan had faded and he had lost some weight. He had the look of a man who had been to the edge, looked over, and decided not to jump.

He was sober.

Bud had come perilously close to killing himself with alcohol, but in the critical moment approaching self-destruction, his psychologist orchestrated an intervention. Bud entered a recovery and rehabilitation program, joined Alcoholics Anonymous, and was rescued from alcoholic meltdown.

That was sixteen years ago. Since then, he has completed a master's in psychology and has become a successful drug and alcohol counselor. Retired from teaching history and mentoring aspiring teachers, he has dedicated his life to helping alcoholics understand their addiction and to learn to find contentment in an increasingly psychotic world; he wants to help save them from certain destruction. He mentored me. Previously unaware of my drinking problem, he heard a lot about my past life once I quit for good. With the unique perspective of a recovering alcoholic psychologist, Bud had many answers to help me understand the dynamics of my alcoholism.

Bud was born into a lower-middle-class, blue-collar family in the early 1940s. His dad was a mechanic, his mother a stay-at-home mom. Neither was highly educated or emotionally mature. His was a "no talk" family. Bud described it as one of those households with an elephant in the living room. A casual observer would take one look at the family interaction and say, "What are you doing with that elephant in the living room?" and everybody in the family would say, "What elephant?" Denial and inability to express emotions characterized this quiet, depressed, and angry household.

In the second grade, Bud went on a class field trip to his first play, *The Emperor's New Clothes*. It was an epiphany. He saw the beauty of the costumes, the complexity of the story, and the pageantry of a stage production and was captivated. A door had been opened on his dark, narrow existence, and Bud immediately fell in love with performance art.

The experience motivated him to read classics such as Dante's *Inferno* and *A Streetcar Named Desire*. He emptied the shelves of the local library, but his extracurricular reading didn't make him a good student. At his high school there was no incentive to achieve and teachers didn't care as long as their students weren't fighting. For Bud, there was no life outside of Norwalk. Working after school as an apprentice mechanic in spite of a burgeoning intellect, Bud prepared for a life in his father's image.

In February of 1958, Bud had another awakening. He didn't want to follow his fellow students to prison or make any life-altering mistakes. He had been dating a "sleazy" girl with sexual experience. One night they "borrowed" a car and some liquor and got really drunk. Bud woke up the next morning to the realization that he may have ruined his life. He recognized that alcohol made him do things he didn't want to do and he swore it off. He dropped the girl and his hoodlum friends and searched for a way out of his lifestyle.

He found her on a sunny beach one Sunday. Her name was Nellie and she came from an impoverished and rigid Lutheran background. Nellie's father was disabled and unable to care for his family. His children were farmed out to relatives. Nellie, at fifteen, was working as a live-in maid for a cousin. She wasn't supposed to be on the beach that Sunday, as recreation on the Sabbath was a sin. But she was. And so was Bud. And in a brief flirtation, each recognized in the other an ally, someone who could help the other get out of the dark, dead-end life each was living. Bud calls it the "Hansel and Gretel" myth: two children lost in the deep dark forest forge a partnership to escape.

Bud took Nellie to the theater and gave her a piece of his dream.

They started dating. Bud flourished in the comfortable, accepting, low-stress relationship. In the light of Nellie's love, he could see a future outside of Norwalk. For Nellie's part, she desired a way out of the poverty and the cultural straitjacket in which she was trapped. Bud was the answer.

The first ever in his family to seek a degree, Bud had enrolled at Cerritos Junior College, but the same inertia he had in high school followed him there. Then, with the advent of Nellie, they both recognized that Bud's intellect could be the vehicle to rescue them from the economic and cultural desert in which they were lost.

Bud's grades soared with his spirits. His partnership with Nellie gave him the motivation to achieve, and he completed his two years at Cerritos with academic honors. Bud and Nellie were married. Given Nellie's Lutheran background and Bud's aversion to alcohol, it was a dry wedding. As Bud and Nellie left the reception, he saw his father pouring himself a drink. Later, they heard from friends and relatives alike that their reception was the most raucous party any had been to in years. Apparently his father offered one of Nellie's uncles a drink. He accepted. Lutherans don't drink often, but before long most of the relatives were imbibing and the party lasted long into the night. One staunch cousin, infuriated at his weak relatives' sinfulness, left the reception and walked two hours to get home.

As Bud gained success, he developed an intellectual and cultural inferiority complex. He knew he had the brains and the work ethic to make it out of his social prison but felt he was entering realms in which he truly did not belong. Searching for four-year schools to complete his degree, he found many prestigious colleges courting him. During the early sixties, social egalitarianism was sweeping the country as the civil rights movement made headlines almost daily. Bud remembers vividly an interview he had at one of the Claremont colleges, renowned bastions of social and educational excellence. As he walked into the foyer of the administration building, he encountered a stunningly beautiful young lady in formal attire playing magnificently on a grand piano. It was as if the starving street urchin had watched a Christmas feast from the window. Bud was impressed, but he felt uncomfortable in such high-class company. He accepted admission at Cal State-Fullerton, a campus of the burgeoning California State College system.

Even at a state college, the mechanic's son from the blue-collar neighborhood felt increasing tension. Bud was rising well above his prior social station, and the fear of entering a forbidden intellectual province, coupled with the hard work of balancing studies with a number of part-time jobs, left Bud highly anxious. After studying at night, he could not sleep. So, he began to drink.

Why would a smart young man who recognized that he was out of control when he drank resort to alcohol to calm his nerves and permit sleep? Out of perceived necessity, and because one of the subtle seductions of alcohol is that he felt he could handle it. The transition from a few drinks to "relax" to hard-core alcoholism is so slow and subtle that it is rarely noticed. But the need was there for Bud. Ignoring the warnings of his past experience, he relied on liquor to help him cope.

At first it was beer. But the sheer volume of beer he had to drink to produce somnolence was daunting. In relatively short order, beer gave way to wine, and then wine gave way to hard liquor, as it required the smallest volume for the best and fastest effect. Each night, Bud would literally drink himself to sleep.

With his hopes combined with those of his beloved Nellie riding on his shoulders, Bud felt the burden. Sixteen-hour days of study and work ended at 10 PM when Bud cracked the whiskey bottle open. After three stiff shots, he would tumble senseless into bed.

As any neurologist will attest, this is not restful sleep. Alcohol produces sleep by depressing the nervous system, a narcosis similar to general anesthesia greatly reducing normal brain activity. But normal brain activity is vital to healthy sleep. The brain functions in a very complex manner during sleep, cycling from states of deep restful sleep to vivid dreaming states associated with rapid eye movement (REM sleep) and back again all night. Each of these sleep states, especially the REM stage, is essential to renew normal healthy brain function. In sleep lab experiments, people who are deliberately awakened each time they approach the REM stage, effectively preventing that stage, progressively develop serious emotional disorders, which may eventuate in frank psychosis.

Unknowingly, Bud was preventing himself from getting the rest he needed. The stupor of alcohol is not the restful sleep of sobriety. The anxiety and the tension in his life were exacerbated by the alcohol-induced sleep. Feeling tired and stressed all the time, Bud responded by drinking more.

And so it went. Bud drank his way through college at Cal State-Fullerton and on to graduate school for his PhD in history at the University of Georgia. It is a tribute to Bud's intellect and to his determination that, in spite of his drinking, he accomplished so much. Aiding in his success was his discovery that vigorous exercise was a great stress releaser as well. Bud was a good athlete and physical activity came easily to him. He began to run, cycle, and swim. In spite of his drinking, he became extremely fit and experienced the endorphin high that is the natural reward of sustained intense physical activity. Between the exercise and the booze, Bud was just able to cope. Barely.

Bud couldn't escape his torment, the constant feeling that he was being judged. He desperately wanted to be part of the world he aspired to: a college professor and aficionado of fine art, music, and drama. He possessed the intellect and the work ethic, but the tension of feeling like an outsider was enormous. He couldn't avoid the fear that his professors and peers would discover he was the blue-collar urchin he was inside. The "Impostor Syndrome" is surprisingly common. Though talented and bright, he believed he was aspiring to something he didn't deserve, going someplace he had no right to be. And he was sure that the guardians of the status quo would find him out and expose him for the fraud he really was.

And so, Bud drank. As his tolerance increased, he began to drink during the day. As he did, gradually, his performance deteriorated. And with time, as he will admit, his morality deteriorated as well. He began to hide how much he drank from Nellie and from his colleagues.

It was a fifteen-year process, the insidious downward spiral: more liquor, lower-quality work, more guilt, more anxiety, more liquor. Without realizing it, Bud had become a hard-core alcoholic. He would wake up shaky and drink to quiet the tremors. And with each passing month, it took more whiskey to calm those shakes, more whiskey to quiet those fears. It was a nightmare. He couldn't live with alcohol, and he couldn't live without it.

I saw Bud as a patient for a year or so during this terrible time. I recall smelling the strong odor of alcohol on his breath and observing intoxicated behavior, wondering if his wife knew how serious his drinking was and wondering how long he could continue with such an obvious problem.

There have been times in my practice when I observed patients coming visit after visit, clearly intoxicated. Somehow, they function drunk for years without dying of liver disease or getting arrested for drunk driving. They reach some kind of alcoholic equilibrium where their behavior, their alcohol intake, and their luck remain the same. This was not so with Bud. His drinking continued to increase as his life approached the brink of crisis. He drank so much he could no longer train, losing the endorphin high that had sustained him for many years. He was at the breaking point.

Nellie was in denial about the severity of Bud's alcoholism. She knew he drank heavily, but she would not confront him since it might jeopardize their future. It was too painful to remember the menial jobs of her childhood. Bud was her white knight, who drank to cope.

On the verge of self-destruction, drinking two quarts of whiskey a day, Bud was referred to a therapist by a friend. Perhaps sensing imminent disaster, Bud went to counseling. Six times. At the end of the sixth visit, the therapist told Bud there was nothing wrong with him; he was simply a liar and a drunk.

The therapist's comment hit Bud like a slap in the face. He could no longer deny it; he was a hopeless drunk. And he knew he was killing himself.

His therapist engineered an intervention. Bud was confronted by his loved ones and coerced into a treatment center in Monterey. Shortly after arrival, he entered the delirium tremens (D.T.s); suddenly withdrawn from a drug he had abused every day for the last twenty-five years, Bud was close to death. He had high fevers and cold sweats. He hallucinated. He had seizures. He was so sick that the staff suggested sending him to the local community hospital, but the center's doctor refused, convinced they were no better equipped to treat Bud's crisis than he was. They wouldn't know there existed a fine human being, a person worth salvaging, inside the pathetic and tragic figure Bud had become. The doctor won. After many long nights, the crisis passed and Bud recovered. He spent thirty-five days in the Monterey Center and was discharged fully detoxed. He was clean and sober but returned to the same environment with the same fears and shame, a situation portending failure. Realizing that he needed some time to work out changes in his life, Bud was able to convince his department head to grant him three months of disability. He spent them at the Alano Club learning how not to drink.

For three months, Bud went to AA meetings, sometimes three and four a day. He acknowledged his addiction and he learned from others like him not to make excuses and to rebuild a life without alcohol. This was the practical side of his recovery, the nuts and bolts of being sober. But the AA concept of "one day at a time" drove him nuts. He acknowledged that the minute-to-minute decision not to drink is what would save him, but his psyche required the long view of life. He needed to see his life in terms of continuous long-lasting sobriety. He needed to better understand the complexity of his personality, the needs that had nearly driven him to oblivion. For that, he turned to therapy. For Bud, they went hand in hand: AA providing the practical solution, therapy supplying the intellectual. For sobriety, there were meetings. For sanity, there was his therapist.

Bud's keen mind began to marvel at the insights he discovered about himself, about addiction, and about getting healthy. The natural result was a master's in psychology and a license in family and marriage counseling. He gradually wound down his teaching career as his psychology practice grew. His forte, of course, is substance abuse. What better qualifications could he have than the twenty-five years of alcoholism he has lived? He knows every excuse, used them each more than once. He's used every rationalization imaginable, fooling almost everyone but himself. He can see through the smoke screen of BS that most alcoholics hide behind. There's no hiding from Bud. He's been there before.

If the patient has any desire to discover the truth and to save himself, Bud has answers to start him on his way. He has done dozens of interventions like the one that ultimately saved him. He knows how to put the two together, the practical and the intellectual—to get the person sober but to give insight into the personality flaws that have led to this circumstance.

He doesn't always succeed, but not from lack of knowledge and commitment. He feels his work is both an obligation and a privilege. He is grateful to be alive, and he knows that Alcoholics Anonymous is not enough. Unless he can give his patient strategies for coping, insight into why the addiction occurred, and a love of the sober person they have within, he can't effect a long-term recovery. Otherwise, it's day-to-day sobriety: habits without understanding. With only half the answer, the relapse rate is frightening.

When Bud got sober, he came back to see me as a patient. His honesty was disarming. Fascinated with the insights he had into the problem, I was in awe of the courage it took to do what he had done. Even then, sixteen years ago, I didn't like the control alcohol had over me. I was ashamed of my weakness and I knew that I needed alcohol too much. But I was powerless to change back then. I never let on to Bud that I had a problem. I just listened to him explain his growth through the recovery process. I listened to him describe the lives of hopelessness some of his patients endured and acknowledged by my agreement that alcohol was a huge problem for many people. But I never admitted that I was one of them.

Bud was my mentor. Once a quarter we would have coffee in the early morning and talk about life. We talked about spiritual growth and the challenges of being an honest person in a world that doesn't honor integrity as much as cleverness. We talked about how we could remain beacons of virtue in a sea of immorality. We agreed that when the society that worships money and power finally self-destructs, we might be able to preserve a tiny bit of the culture and save it for the renaissance. And we were both certain that we needed each other and like-minded souls to keep the light alive. Additionally, we agreed that it was enough if we could save one soul at a time. And all along, I secretly knew that I couldn't be true to the righteousness that I aspired to as long as I was drinking. It was similar to discovering I couldn't run any better while I was still smoking. When running became important enough, I quit the smoking. I knew that when the spiritual need grew great enough, I would quit drinking. But, in spite of the fact that I had beaten other addictions (amphetamines and cigarettes), I could not find within me the strength I needed to quit. Looking back, I realize it was because I was not completely committed spiritually. I could still hold back a little, be Jeff Herten, in control of my life and my drinking. I could quit anytime I wanted. I was the boss and I had the strength. But as the years rolled by, I was still drinking. I was not totally committed, and there was an emptiness in my heart. One day I realized I was strong, but not strong enough to quit. I needed more strength than I had. I needed God. When I finally surrendered, allowed myself to be filled with the Holy Spirit, I couldn't drink anymore. They were diametrically opposed.

When I quit, it was a joy to tell Bud about it. Now, I am completely honest with him, completely in agreement on how drinking costs a person his soul. We still have coffee together, but now there is nothing but the truth between us. I love the person that I have become sober, I revel in the strength that it took for me to quit, and I thank God daily for that strength and for saving my life.

Fortunately for me, I didn't have to drink to the brink of oblivion like Bud did to finally quit. I quit when I realized I was powerless to quit alone. That awareness made all the difference.

22

WHO'S FOOLING WHOM? CONCEALING THE PROBLEM

The neurologists were puzzled. Colin Murphy had a severe and progressive neurological disease with profound muscle weakness and loss of coordination, which had developed three months prior. Not the typical profile for multiple sclerosis or Lou Gehrig's disease, Colin was a mystery until the neurologists requested a dermatology consult and I was called. The patient had peculiar white bands extending horizontally across all of his finger and toenails. It was Mee's lines: the classical clinical picture of arsenic poisoning. I took the supervising neurologist aside and explained the diagnosis. A twenty-four-hour urine for heavy metals confirmed my suspicion, and within two weeks, Colin's wife had been arrested and the patient was dramatically better.

It's remarkable how much a trained observer can learn from looking at the skin. I was blessed with good powers of observation and a curious nature. These skills have served me well as a clinical dermatologist. Like Mee's lines, the skin presents innumerable signs of a patient's lifestyle and general health and truly is a window into the individual's physical and emotional life. Something as seemingly trivial as slight bluish discoloration of the fingernails with nearly imperceptible swelling of the last digit might indicate a grave lung condition. An irregular narrowing of a hair shaft may reveal a serious eating disorder. Because of my personal history with alcohol, I am particularly sensitive to the many skin signs of alcohol abuse. Twenty percent of the adult patients in my practice reveal a significant use of, if not a problem with, alcohol.

Howard is a sixty-something semiretired educator with fair skin who sees me regularly for skin cancer problems. He likes early-morning appointments, so I see him between 7 and 8 AM twice a year. More often than not, he has the smell of alcohol on his breath. He has very fair skin with the crimson cheeks of his northern European heritage, and they are especially flushed when I see him for his early-morning visits. I am sure he is not aware that I can detect alcohol on his breath at 7 AM, denoting he has already been drinking or that he is still off-gassing ethanol from a serious bout of drinking the night before. Howard's wife sees me at six-month intervals as well. Her visits are in the afternoon, and I have never noted alcohol on her breath or observed any of the stigmata of alcohol abuse.

Warren was a seventy-or-so entrepreneur, a big man who was also obese. He had massive swelling of his parotid glands overlying his jaw on both sides, blocking the lower half of his ears from view. He suffered hardening of the arteries from years of cigarette smoking, and diabetes and high blood pressure from overindulgence in food and in whiskey. Parotid swelling is a hallmark of the hard drinker. The alcohol, functioning as a sugar and contributing to the obesity, played a role in producing the diabetes as well. Warren would show up for early-morning appointments with alcohol on his breath. He recently died of the complications of diabetes and arteriosclerosis, still drinking at the end.

Carla is a late-forties mother of two going through a nasty divorce. She is frankly tipsy and reeking of alcohol at her early-afternoon appointment.

John is a late-forties disabled highway worker for the state. He has a legitimate skin condition from the stress of an overbearing and dictatorial boss but claims that the pain it causes requires prescription narcotics. He has been cited several times for attempting to fill the same prescription twice before refills were needed. He, too, prefers early-morning appointments and has the smell of alcohol on his breath.

Larry is a mid-fifties businessman who struggles to satisfy a high-maintenance wife. During the last five years, I have noticed the capillaries on his face becoming more livid and the puffiness around his eyes more prominent. Larry drinks too much.

Dorothy was a hard-core alcoholic. Over the last ten years, I watched as her skin became more sallow, and she developed the large spider hemangiomas that indicate impending liver failure. Next her belly grew big as an enlarged, alcoholic liver protruded beneath her rib cage. Then, the liver shrank as it scarred and the big belly was caused by ascites, a fluid that weeps from the scarred and failing liver and builds up in the abdomen. The last time I saw Dorothy, she had a coarse tremor that may have been a "liver flap," another sign of impending failure as ammonia, usually detoxified by the liver, builds up in the bloodstream and the brain. She had one gastrointestinal bleed, from alcoholic gastritis, and her doctor warned her that she had to stop drinking or it would kill her. It did when her liver and kidneys failed. The mortality rate of this condition, known as hepatorenal syndrome, is extremely high.

In medical school, students are taught to do a thorough history and physical examination. The history is a multipart record of the present illness, family history, past illnesses and surgeries, medications, review of all the systems, and a social history. Important facts in this section are marital status, job, children, and use of tobacco, alcohol, and "social" drugs such as marijuana, cocaine, heroin, and so on. Since these medical records can be requested by insurance companies, attorneys, and law enforcement, you can imagine that some of the responses to the latter questions may be less than completely candid.

As a medical student, I was taught that whatever quantity of alcohol consumption a patient admits to, the truth is probably twice that—or more. If the patient says he drinks two beers a night, it is probably four or five. If he admits to two glasses of wine with dinner, he and his wife probably polish off a bottle together. People generally are embarrassed to admit how much they drink, so they naturally decrease the true amount. There are obvious exceptions: people who totally abstain are often vehement about it and they can be trusted. Some alcoholics completely deny imbibing, but the evidence of their dishonesty is displayed all over their bodies. With time, a clever interviewer can spot the inconsistency between the history and the physical findings.

On the other hand, some heavy drinkers and frank alcoholics are quite honest about how much they drink. They will candidly report that they drink a twelve-pack of beer (or more) a night, or a fifth of bourbon, or a bottle and a half of wine. Some are curiously proud of their accomplishment.

Recovering alcoholics are usually quite honest about their past abuse, and it is astonishing to learn how much a person can drink and not die, at least in the short term.

There is cryptic shorthand that doctors use to identify the drinking habits of their patients. It developed long before there was concern that medical records were "discoverable" by attorneys and might end up in court, before all the current concern about the privacy of a patient's medical record. It was just a coded way for the physician to record his observations in the patient's chart without it being obvious to someone other than another doctor.

Interesting notations show up in the margin or the text of the chart note for that visit. "HBD" in the margin of the chart stood for "has been drinking." "ETOH" was a less subtle notation, representing an abbreviation for ethanol, the chemical name for ethyl alcohol. Another surreptitious way of documenting such observations would be to write "Two-carbon disease," as alcohol is a two-carbon molecule. "2-C problem" is another and perhaps even more obscure way to record the obvious signs of alcoholism in a patient without creating an easily understandable note for the office staff or the insurance claims person who might read the patient's chart.

In recent years, some of my colleagues have become less charitable. On the problem list heading the patient's chart is "Problem 3: Alcohol abuse." Bear in mind that the American Psychiatric Association defines alcohol abuse as drinking one or more drinks three times a week. That doesn't leave many out, does it? I often wondered how plaintiffs' attorneys handle these chart note entries in court. Say the patient is suing for complications that occurred after a surgery, perhaps a wound infection. The notation of "alcohol abuse" is a social stigma for the patient, and the common medical knowledge that alcohol suppresses the immune system and increases the potential for infection would make pursuing this suit difficult at best, especially before a jury.

As a young physician, I never felt comfortable frankly confronting patients' alcohol habits. I observed and recorded the progressive signs of liver damage and failure on Dorothy's chart, but I never mentioned it to her. Partly I was embarrassed to bring it up and partly, as a high-functioning alcoholic, I felt I didn't have the right to judge my patients. Now sober, I still try not to judge my alcoholic patients because I see alcohol addiction as a disease and not a character disorder, but I try to help patients become aware that they have a bigger problem than they realize.

Last week, Tom, a mid-forties businessman, was in the office for an exam. He had all the signs of heavy drinking: puffiness around the eyes, coarse dilated capillaries over his nose, a fine tremor, and several new spiders on his face and upper back. I have noticed alcohol on his breath several times in past visits. Not all spiders are signs of severe liver problems. They occur normally in fair-skinned people, in young adolescent females on oral contraceptives, and in pregnancy. But adding it all up, I decided that perhaps Tom needed to know that his alcoholism was taking a toll. I pointed out one of the spiders and asked how long it had been there. Six months, he responded. He inquired what caused them. Well, I said, sometimes they just happen, while at other times, they may be an indication of internal problems. What kind of internal problems? he asked. Well, I am sure this doesn't apply to you, I said, but sometimes they are the sign of early liver damage from drinking. But you don't drink that much, do you? I ask. Not that much, he replied. I drink a couple of beers a night (translation: at least a six-pack). His concern is way out of proportion for someone who really drinks two beers a night. That's not enough to cause spiders, I said. Sometimes these just occur in fair-skinned people and that's probably the answer. He wouldn't let it go. How does drinking cause spiders? he asked. Again, I assured him that this couldn't apply to him but explained that in heavy drinkers the damaged liver can't break down estrogens and that higher levels of circulating estrogens cause the spiders. But don't worry, I said. If it were really from liver damage, you'd notice other things. Like what? he asked. Well, the increased estrogen causes the testicles to shrivel up. Makes you impotent, I offered. I watched his pupils get large; it was obvious that I had his attention. You don't have any problems like that? I asked. No, he lied. The greatest shame for a man is not functioning sexually, so I'm not surprised he denied it. The look of concern was written on his face. I had scored a direct hit, but he tried not to let on. He asked me, in the abstract, if there's any way to treat or repair the liver damage. It's pretty far advanced at that point, I offered, but the liver is an amazingly resilient organ and some repair is possible, if the drinker abstains. We ended the visit with Tom still trying to ask questions and with me reassuring him that couldn't be the problem by his drinking history. Tom is a hypochondriac and perhaps his anxiety over health concerns will force him to face his alcohol problem. I had been honest with him. Perhaps I had an impact.

Physicians sometimes make critical errors in not realizing how heavily their patients drink. A well-respected judge who alleges to drinking "a glass" of wine at dinner had an abnormal liver function test. This prompted the physician to do an expensive and fruitless workup for hepatitis and rare liver diseases when the problem is that the judge drinks too much. I saw a case recently of a prominent local businessman who repeatedly had elevated liver enzymes. The clinician did an exhaustive workup and found nothing, yet every time he checked the patient's blood, those same liver enzymes were elevated. As a result, the doctor scheduled a liver biopsy, not the most benign procedure. A long, large gauge needle is inserted in the patient's right mid back, aiming for the liver. Done correctly, a small core sample of liver is recovered. With poor or unlucky aim, a large artery in the liver might be punctured or lacerated, causing massive bleeding. Occasionally, the lower edge of the chest cavity is penetrated and the patient suffers a pneumothorax or punctured lung. As a pathology resident, I interpreted liver biopsies and occasionally a piece of kidney was all that was recovered from the needle. Suffice it to say that a liver biopsy is not an entirely safe procedure. I treat patients with psoriasis with a medication that is toxic to the liver, and periodic liver biopsies are mandatory to ensure that the patient is not progressing to cirrhosis. When I request one, the gastroenterologist always makes me insist that I really need it, because he doesn't like performing them. So this really high-risk biopsy is being done on a patient to assess his liver when the real problem is that he drinks a liter of wine every night. But the judge and his doctor never had an honest conversation about how much he was really drinking, nor did the doctor insist that he abstain for a week or two before repeating the liver enzymes. Knowing both the doctor and the patient well, I was astounded that they had never had that conversation. Before I submit my patient to a liver biopsy, I certainly would.

With hard-core alcoholics, information and education about the progression of their liver disease does no good. They are out of control and literally not able to stop once they start drinking until they pass out. But they have heard the words; they know the negative consequences of their addiction.

There is a saying among recovering alcoholics: the alcoholic is the last one to know. It's true. The spouse knows, the boss knows, coworkers know, the children know, friends know. The trashman who empties five empty vodka bottles a week knows. The doctor knows. But cunning, baffling, powerful alcohol masks the truth from the drinker until the very end. Then, the inexorable progression of the disease takes its toll.

23

JACK MCDOUGALL: THE DRUNK IN THE CORPORATE BOARDROOM

When I was growing up, my parents had a large and interesting circle of friends. Many factors bound them together. The women belonged to several volunteer organizations. Most of the group played golf, all were upper-middle-class, and to a person, they all drank.

I was fascinated by Jack McDougall, a member of the group. An enormously successful realtor, Jack was chairman of the board of the second largest real estate firm in the nation. He took it public when I was in my twenties, realizing tens of millions of dollars in stock. But if you met Jack at a barbecue or party, you'd never guess he was a shrewd, successful businessman. He looked, talked, and drank like an old cowboy.

Jack grew up in McKittrick, California, a bleak little town on the west side of the San Joaquin Valley, most notable for its large deposits of oil. He grew up riding horses and doing hard physical work, went to UC-Berkeley, worked for a time for the IRS, and then found that his Will Rogers persona and his financial aspirations were ideal for the real estate business. What's more, in all his endeavors, Jack found he had a secret weapon, an advantage over his clients and the competition. Jack McDougall could drink vast quantities and function at a very high level.

To enhance his image, Jack rolled his own cigarettes, a throwback to his old wrangler days. It was enthralling to watch him pull a little cloth sack of tobacco out of his shirt pocket, pour it with one hand onto a cigarette paper, close the purse string of the pouch with his teeth, curl the paper to concentrate the tobacco, lick the edge, and expertly roll a stubby but firm cigarette.

I would watch Jack with fascination when he came to our home for a dinner party. He matched my dad drink for drink before dinner. This warm-up consisted of two or three hard liquor drinks. With dinner there was wine. With dessert, they drank Kahlua, Galliano, or brandy. And then, when the party stretched into the wee hours, Jack would switch to beer. Looking back, I am astounded at the volume of alcohol that was consumed. Jack's consumption equaled anyone's, but I never saw him drunk. He would just stand there with his shoulders set at a confident angle, cigarette in his left hand, his right hand gesturing to make a point, his weather-beaten face accented by clear and observant eyes. A very smart man, he exuded a quiet confidence, but never arrogance.

Jack McDougall knew how to use that intelligence, his very personable social skills, and his ability to drink to rise to the top of the real estate business. He was as comfortable in the locker rooms of the most exclusive country clubs as he was on a horse. At work, Jack reportedly kept a fifth of bourbon and several glasses on the sideboard in his office. It was his secretary's responsibility to replace it with a full one daily. And each day, usually with some help from clients and business partners, that bottle would be empty by quitting time. Negotiations were undertaken over a drink. Contracts were signed and deals were sealed with a handshake and a drink. And when the bargaining got tense and heated, the coolest man in the room, with the highest blood alcohol, was Jack McDougall. How many bargains did he strike intoxicated? How many concessions and compromises did he gain because he was able to hold his liquor better than his adversary?

Lots.

Jack once told me that he only did business two days a week: Tuesday and Thursday. When I looked startled, he explained.

"Jeff, you never try to make a deal on Monday. Your customer just got back from a weekend at the lake and his mind is still there. On Wednesday, he plays golf in the afternoon, so his mind isn't on business in the morning. On Friday, he's getting ready to go away for the weekend and his mind is already there. So you never call him those days. Tuesdays and Thursdays—that's when I do all my business."

Of course, he was right. Jack figured it all out early in his career and used it to his advantage.

In his later years, Jack's cancerous larynx was removed. He used a small handheld silver amplifier to squawk out short responses. Mouth and throat cancer have two major predisposing factors: tobacco and alcohol. The doctors at his alma mater were miraculously able to save him, and he lived to a ripe late-eighties, croaking with his silver amplifier and smiling that wry smile.

I can imagine you're wondering, what's wrong with the way he lived? He was fabulously successful and respected in the business community, and he had raised a family, enjoyed life, and lived into old age. What's wrong with that?

Nothing, if you agree that Jack McDougall alone did not do all those things. It was not Jack that made the money, raised those kids, and enjoyed those rodeos. It was Jack and alcohol. It was Jack fortified with whiskey.

So what? So alcohol was a crutch, a coping mechanism, a tool Jack McDougall used to function successfully in his world. It calmed his nerves while he negotiated the big deals and eased his social anxiety at big board meetings. It gave him that competitive edge working in the world of high finance. It made him feel good.

What if his drug of choice had been heroin? What if it had been crack cocaine or crystal meth? Would that have been okay? Why is one drug, alcohol, socially acceptable and another, heroin, not? Why is the person addicted to cocaine treated as a pariah, while the person addicted to alcohol is revered and emulated? Because alcohol is legal? There is a disconnect here in our social consciousness. If Jack had landed in the gutter, his alcoholism may have been viewed as a problem. In the plush boardrooms of the Fortune 500, it is not.

Why not?

Alcohol, although legal, is a drug, and Jack is an addict.

There's a story about a man who meets a woman in a bar and asks her to sleep with him for a hundred dollars. She refuses, saying, "What do you think I am, a prostitute?" He is a very wealthy man, so he pulls out his checkbook, writes a check for fifty thousand dollars, and hands it to the lady. She follows him to his room. Afterward, he says to her, "Lady, we're not arguing about what you are or aren't. We're just haggling over the price."

We're not arguing over whether or not Jack McDougall was a drug addict. He was. We're just arguing that the drug he became addicted to does not carry the social stigma of heroin or crack cocaine.

The important point is that Jack didn't need alcohol to climb the ladder of success. If he could do it drunk, he could do it better sober. He had the right stuff in him. He just didn't think he could. When deprived of their chemical coping mechanism, some people are convinced they can't function. The truth is they can and will function as well or better if they find strength elsewhere in their lives.

I have a touch of stage fright. In spite of forty years of public speaking experience, debating and teaching at the regional and national level in dermatology and dermatopathology, I still get butterflies and more than a little tightness in my chest when the lights go down and I am at the podium with two or three hundred people watching. In my early teaching days, there were times I would have a couple of beers half an hour before my lecture. They would relax me just enough to get me started and take the edge off my anxiety.

When I quit drinking, I didn't quit teaching or public speaking. But now, sober, I summon the strength it took me to quit, and that, rather than two beers, sees me through. I have never been calmer and more clearheaded in my presentations than I have been since becoming sober.

The first step on the road to sobriety is to acknowledge that you are powerless to control your drinking and to seek a higher power that will give you the strength to quit. You do not have to name this higher power. It is whatever you find within yourself that is strong enough to overcome the addiction.

For me, that power is God. I had been a practicing Christian for many years, but my actions and my drinking revealed that I hadn't put all my faith and trust in him since I still needed alcohol to cope. I was addicted to alcohol. I needed it to deal with the long hours, the hard schedule, and the anxiety of work. I hated what it did to me, but I couldn't quit. I had more faith in alcohol to get me through than I did in God. There is a Scripture verse that states you cannot serve two masters; you must choose whom you would serve. I was giving lip service to God and worshipping Budweiser. When I was finally ready, I prayed that God would give me the strength to quit. And I promised to serve only Him.

After five years, I have kept my promise and He has kept his. I am sober and every day I give thanks that I am no longer a slave to alcohol.

If Jack McDougall could succeed brilliantly in real estate intoxicated, whatever he needed was already within him. I now lean on God, not alcohol, to get me through the difficult times. I am much stronger than I had ever imagined I could be. My shame is gone. I love the person that I have become, the real Jeff Herten, not the Jeff Herten fortified with three beers.

I look back in wonder at the change in me. I hated my previous lack of control and the power that alcohol had over me. I have enormous empathy for people who are completely lost in alcohol: for the helplessness and the worthlessness they feel. I remember meeting Bill at a men's social trail ride ten years ago. A big man with huge hands and a soft handshake, he was a hunter, a collector of rare rifles and shotguns, and a very gentle and kind man. I watched with great respect as he drank soft drinks for four days, while the two hundred "wannabe" cowboys drank themselves silly. He was a recovering alcoholic, he explained, and he seemed to have no difficulty abstaining. I was in awe of his discipline, but a mutual friend later explained that if Bill took a drink he would not stop until he passed out and that he had been in and out of alcohol rehab programs three times. Currently, he had been dry for over six months. A few months later, his obituary appeared in our local paper. I contacted a mutual friend and learned that Bill had lost his battle with alcohol. Feeling hopeless against his addiction, Bill put the barrel of a shotgun in his mouth and pulled the trigger.

Suicide is not an uncommon fate for those who feel hopelessly addicted. Unable to believe they'll ever beat it, they give up. Former Boston Celtic Larry Bird knows the story all too well. He was raised in abject poverty in rural Indiana, chiefly because his father could never make it home with a paycheck. He was a serious drunk, and it was Larry's mom who saved the family from total disintegration. When Larry was in high school, his dad could no longer handle the hopelessness and shame and killed himself.

My acquaintance Bill and Larry Bird's dad are extreme examples of the destructive potential of alcohol. Most drinkers have only moderate disruptions to their lives from alcohol and continue drinking. Many are just "social drinkers" until there's a life crisis or a bout of depression and consequently they become problem drinkers. Some reading this book may feel smug because they think they don't have a problem. If you really think that your drinking is not a problem, turn to chapter 34 and honestly answer its questions.

24

ERNEST HEMINGWAY: THE MAN'S MAN AND THE DRUNK'S DRUNK

○ ○

"The bartender placed two frozen daiquiris in front of us; they were in conical glasses twice the size of my previous drink. 'Here we have the ultimate achievement of the daiquiri-maker's art,' Hemingway said. 'Made a run of sixteen here one night.'
'This size?'
'House record,' the barman, who had been listening, said.
Hemingway sampled his drink by taking a large mouthful, holding it for a long moment, then swallowing it in several installments. He nodded approval."

Havana, 1948
From Papa Hemingway, by A.E. Hotchner

He could say more with fewer words than any other author. He captured the beauty and emotion of a scene like few others I have ever read. As a young writer, he would spend days honing a two-page description of a scene into a single paragraph. He said that what you left out was more important than what you put in. When reading his novels, one has to imagine his intent at times. It is these mysterious omissions that make his writing so engaging. Ernest Hemingway, Nobel

Prize winner and one of the greatest writers of the twentieth century, struggled with alcoholism all his life, and it coauthored his demise.

He was born into the upper middle class, in a wealthy suburb of Chicago, the son of a doctor who committed suicide at an early age. As a boy, Hemingway's summers in the Upper Peninsula of Michigan left him with a lifelong love of fishing, hunting, and the rugged self-reliance of the outdoorsman. He left his home and country to drive an ambulance in Italy in World War I and then lived in Paris, joining a group of self-exiled American artists that included Ezra Pound and Gertrude Stein. And he wrote. And he drank.

Hemingway was obsessed with masculinity. He boxed, wrestled, brawled, hunted, fished, and drank with gusto. He fancied himself a great lover, but by all accounts he was mediocre; being rather self-absorbed, it is unlikely that he was interested in pleasuring a partner or that he was sober enough to do so most of the time.

Hemingway suffered "black periods," when he couldn't create and was drinking hard. As he matured, he began to realize that he couldn't drink and write. He would go on the wagon, rise early, write for three or four hours, and rediscover his creative genius. He was physically healthy, lived a Spartan life, and wrote well and prolifically. Some of his greatest literary achievements were accomplished during these periods. Hemingway was always content during these times of creativity and sobriety. Inevitably, however, upon completion of a book, he would begin drinking hard again.

As the years passed and his fame grew, so did the "friends" and hangers-on. Solitude, discipline, and sobriety were harder to achieve. Celebrity brought wealth and more opportunities to travel, hunt, party, and drink. As a result, he began to have difficulty with high blood pressure. The alcoholic calories that expanded his waistline exacerbated his blood pressure problem. The physical deterioration caused by his alcoholism—high blood pressure, failing eyesight, memory loss, poor concentration, and lack of endurance, strength, and sexual prowess—caused severe depression abetted by his enormous alcohol intake.

During the last decade of his life as an aging writer, the Nobel Prize and lucrative movie contracts in hand, he struggled to create for a demanding public. But his physical and mental decline rendered him incapable of his previous genius. He suffered intractable hypertension and obsessively took his blood pressure, logging it in a small book dozens of times a day. Robbed of his discipline and gift of prose, Hemingway's inability to cope created a psychotic depression. The delicate balance of neurotransmitters that determines state of mind had gone tragically awry, in part abetted by years of alcoholism.

And as is so common in the progression of alcoholism, the drinking that had always been able to soothe the depression now magnified it, leading to a failed suicide attempt. The pain had grown too great. There was no hope of regaining his creative genius. Suicide was Hemingway's only solution. One autumn day in Idaho, he put the barrel of a shotgun in his mouth and definitively ended his agony.

The scene is not uncommon: great minds with sacred gifts squandered in a losing battle with alcohol addiction.

We need to make the public more aware that yes, alcohol brings wildly exciting abandonment to pleasure and lack of inhibition, but it also comes with a yoke of dependence that for many is difficult or impossible to shed. The short-term glamour, excitement, and sexiness of alcohol may be replaced with physical and psychological addiction and a depression that few are able to tolerate. With the immersion of our culture in the media blitz created by the alcohol industry, this is a daunting challenge. Perhaps by telling our stories and those tragedies like Ernest Hemingway's, we can open eyes and minds to the peril.

25

PRIDE COMETH BEFORE THE DRINK

◆

The failure of personal strength and willpower in the battle against alcohol

Discipline is my middle name. I'm the guy who never missed a day of running in two years, the guy who got up at 4:30 AM every morning so I could get ten miles in before work, then worked a full day, and then ran five miles after work for months at a time. I quit nail biting. I quit cigarettes. I quit amphetamines. I lost thirty-five pounds on the Atkins diet. Yes sir, I have a will of iron. I could will myself to run the last seventy-five miles of a hundred-mile run with a sprained ankle.

Quit drinking? No problem. I'd quit so many times that I'd lost count. Just one problem: I couldn't maintain it. I'd always start again. Then one day, shamed and humiliated, I wanted to quit more than I ever wanted anything in my life. But I knew I was powerless to do it on my own. So I got down on my knees and I asked God to take this burden, this addiction, off my shoulders.

And he did.

He did what I couldn't do. He led me to sobriety. And as long as I remember that it is through his grace and love that I got sober, through his power and not my own, I can stay sober.

One of the remarkable ironies of alcoholism is that willpower and personal strength often fail in the end. The proud alcoholic, who, like me, truly believes he can quit anytime he wills it, is sadly deluded. Personal strength is a real handicap in the quest for sobriety. It takes years for an arrogant alcoholic like me to come to the awareness that he has a problem, then years more for him to realize that he can't "fix" it himself. By then, he has lost a job or a wife, or both. Perhaps he's had a couple of DUIs or he's hurt someone while driving under the influence. He's lost his temper in a drunken rage and screamed at his children so many times that it's now a learned response in them, and they're likely to treat their kids similarly. Oftentimes, the proud and arrogant person never gets it; he never realizes that alcohol is too "cunning, baffling, and powerful" (Alcoholics Anonymous 2001) to overcome alone. It is a rare individual who is strong enough to achieve sobriety without help from a higher power.

Personal strength alone is not the answer. It didn't work for my friend Kate. She grew up in an alcoholic family and she started drinking after she was raped at the age of thirteen. She stole most of her booze by walking into a liquor store and, when the clerk was occupied with another customer, walking out with a fifth of tequila. No one would suspect a cute thirteen-year-old girl.

Kate drank hard until she was thirty-five. Then, after a near-crippling accident, she experienced a "moment of clarity" that allowed her to see what a mess her life was and how it had all started with alcohol. She quit the same day, summoning all of her personal strength and discarding every bottle she had in the house.

But, Kate didn't seek support to stay sober. She figured she could do it on her own. She didn't get professional help, didn't join AA, and didn't begin the process of identifying the issues that had led her to drink. She was sober but not seeking the understanding and contentment that could keep her sober.

She lasted a little over a year. I planned to relate her experience in detail, but when I sent a draft of her chapter, she fired back a terse note that she didn't want to bare herself, share her story. I wrote back inquiring if she was still sober. There was no reply.

It happens. Alcoholics fall off the wagon—even those who ask God to take over for them. But it happens a lot more often to the alcoholic who fights his addiction alone. He just doesn't have the ammunition to battle such a formidable foe.

Strong-willed sober alcoholics who don't seek support risk becoming "dry drunks." They still have the problems, bad temper, dishonesty, and feelings of guilt and inferiority that they had when drinking. They are sober, yet sobriety has not provided them peace and contentment. Some obsess about alcohol more than when they were drinking. I heard a fellow say that for the three years he was sober, he couldn't get through a day without thinking about alcohol. Finally, when he began drinking again, there was a tremendous sense of relief. He was drinking instead of obsessing about it. He drank for a year before his life became so unmanageable that he accepted rehab again and acknowledged for the first time that he couldn't do it by himself. He surrendered to alcohol. He gave up trying to win a battle that he now knew he could not win alone. Strategic surrender is the road that leads to sobriety and happiness.

Sally's worried face reflected that her son, Rick, was in jail again: another DUI. He had just gotten his license back after two years.

"I know he'll quit this time. He's a very strong person, and if they threaten to put his son in a foster home, I know he can quit."

Probably not.

Rick will quit when he realizes that alcohol is ruining his life, and that he can't quit on his own but needs support to fight this battle. But Rick is proud and he may not get it this time. Surrender takes humility.

Pride and a sense of personal strength also lead many alcoholics to believe that they can drink moderately. They want to be "social drinkers" like other people. The goal of "drinking like a gentleman" has them drinking just at parties on the weekends, for a while. But fairly quickly they are drinking almost every day, and sooner rather than later their lives are out of control again.

What if you don't believe in a higher power? You're unsure that there is a God, so how can you call on Him for help? When you are desperate enough, when you have been humbled and humiliated enough to realize that you can't do it alone, simply ask. It requires a "rigorous honesty" to finally have that moment of truth, to know that there really is no other way. That awareness is truly an unrealized gift from God. He is asking you to let Him help. Suppress your ego and pride and ask for His help. Ask Him to lift this crushing burden from your shoulders.

You may be shocked at the results.

I was. The dark night of hopeless futility suddenly became a brilliant dawn of freedom. It was a miracle, an incredible gift of grace that proved to me there was a God. It proved to me that He loved me and that He wanted me sober.

For that I thank Him daily.

26

HE HAD IT ALL, EXCEPT CONTROL OF HIS DRINKING

I sat in the pew and wept. Three hundred and fifty miles away, they were burying my friend, Pete.

He died in a single-vehicle rollover, ejected and crushed beyond identification.

He was one of the finest men I have known. Ten years my senior, he shared my love of horses. He had been raised with them, scion of a pioneer family with great tradition in our town. Enormously successful, he shared his wealth with the community in countless ways, both seen and unseen. He always had the time and resources to aid the poor and disadvantaged, and most of his generosity and self-lessness went publicly unacknowledged.

He wanted it that way.

He had a smile and a kind word for everyone he met, and a memorable story or two were sure to bring laughter. I always looked forward to our encounters.

Pete had only one fault. He drank too much. There was always a beer in his hand or a pitcher of Bloody Marys beside the barbecue. In many ways, he reminded me of my dad: never drunk but always drinking.

He finished his tennis match that Thursday, had a few with his friends, and was headed home. He misjudged a curve on the coast highway and lost control of his car. In an instant it was over.

The church was filled to overflowing and the eulogies only hinted at the self-lessness and the generosity of the man. I wasn't there. I had a date with a hundred-mile trail over the Sierras that I had been preparing for over a year. I knew Pete would understand. On the day of the ride, I wore a simple yellow ribbon tied around my strong right arm. Pete rode with me that day.

Two weeks after the tragedy, there was a one-paragraph article in the local paper. The victim of the rollover had a blood alcohol of 0.28 percent.

I heard that some friends and family had confronted Pete about his drinking several weeks before his death. He refused to agree there was a problem.

Beyond my sadness and the grief of his family and friends is the tragedy that this truly good man has, for many, left only one memory. They won't remember the untold generosity and altruism.

They only will remember that he died drunk.

27

THE TRAIL RIDE

The front of the trail camp bar was a dangerous place to be. Like a fire hydrant in a neighborhood of male dogs, it had been marked as home territory by every young cowboy in camp. Now that the day's ride was over, they were getting liquored up. The first to stake claim in front was tall and lanky, sinewy arms bulging from a cutoff T-shirt. A worn Stetson pushed back on his head, he sipped tequila from a shot glass and strutted right in front of the bar. Not for long. There was sudden movement. A body hurdled in from the right, cutting him down at mid thigh. A circle of yelling cowboys instantly formed as bodies thrashed in the dirt. Stetson was bigger and stronger, but he was drunk and lacked speed. The smaller man, compact but powerful, was cat-quick and less drunk. Over they went, then back again, the drunken crowd of cowboys shouting advice and derision amid straining muscles, dirt-stained faces, and sweaty shirts. Then a lightning takedown and the challenger was behind him, clutching a leg, driving Stetson into the ground, the trademark hat off now and crumpled in the dust. His college wrestling skills imprinted in muscle memory even after a decade, the challenger strained to turn his larger foe. For a moment there was stalemate, then Stetson, tiring, began to yield ground and the smaller man, sensing the kill, drove him over and was on him like a lion, arm around his neck, smothering him with his arched and straining body.

The crowd roared, "One, two, three," and then howled approval at the pin. Near exhaustion, the two men stood up and shook hands, dusted off their torn clothes, and had yet another beer. And the new king of the bar watched for the next challenger. There would be several more before the afternoon was over.

Indeed, only a fool or someone looking for a fight would stand at the front of the bar. There had been words earlier in the day on the trail. The grizzly-bearded old police sergeant, fortified with a few whiskeys, figured it was time to show that "smart-ass kid" who is boss. Without warning and with surprising quickness, he had a choke hold on the stocky cowboy. He choked him down right there at the bar, leaving him senseless in the dust. As two friends dragged the cowboy away, the old man sipped a few more whiskeys and crowed, "That ought to teach him." An hour later, the stocky cowboy, nursing a sore windpipe, coldcocked the old man, knocking him out. He lay there for a full five minutes, blowing clouds of dust around a small pool of blood. Then he painfully got up and retired to his camp to ice his eye and clean his face. Later that afternoon, I spent an hour sewing up the three-inch split beneath his eye.

The side of the bar was a less dangerous place to be, but on that day the ride had been short and the buckaroos had been back in camp and drinking for several hours, so there was no safe haven. A slight young man visited with friends, unsuspecting, when an old man howled and jumped on his back. Off-balance, the young man fell forward and his attacker, screaming a war whoop, bit him viciously on the back. The biter leaped up and, arms above his head, paraded around in triumph. The drunken crowd screamed approval and the young man, shocked at the violence of his first trail ride, disappeared back to his camp. The biter would strike twice more within the hour, but his third victim was sober and waiting for him. As the biter prepared to leap, his victim handily sidestepped him, raised a leg, and tripped the unsteady attacker, who sprawled face-first in the dirt. The intended victim then sat on him and packed that once-feared mouth with dirt and leaves and left him to pass out in the dust.

The violence at the bar that afternoon had reached an all-time high. Unfortunately the trail boss had planned too short a ride for the day, allowing the cowboys three hours at the bar before the evening barbecue. The black eyes and torn shirts were directly proportional to the additional time spent in front of that now familiar bar.

It happens every spring. Two hundred and fifty-odd ranchers, lawyers, doctors, professors, and assorted businessmen, many of whom had their last ride thirty years ago for a quarter in front of the grocery store, camp with borrowed and leased horses and reenact the glory days of early California history.

"Mount up, boys. It's a trail ride."

Each morning after breakfast, sack lunches on saddles and many fortified with gin fizzes or a few shots at the bar, the buckaroos mount for the day's ride. Loose girths and slipped saddles attest to the greenness of the dudes. Somebody is always bucked off before the column heads out of camp. The trail boss, usually an accomplished horseman, possibly a little more sober than the rest, and hopefully knowledgeable about the route, keeps the men out on the trail (and away from the bar) as long as possible.

Starting and stopping, winding up the trail at a walk, the long line of riders expands and contracts like the dragon at Chinese New Year. The riders pass back and forth canteens and botas filled with schnapps or a deadly recipe called "whistle," part Everclear and part diesel fuel. Forty minutes to an hour is all these tender butts can take. Then, magically, there is a large clearing and two pickups loaded with coolers and the essential liquid: beer.

"Let 'em blow, boys. It's a trail ride," the trail boss says, as if the horses are winded enough to need a rest. But the gluteals of many of the riders certainly do.

The buckaroos mill around the trucks, drawing their ration. A few of the young bucks gallop through the scattered horses, hats off and waving, trying to provoke a stampede. Shade is a premium at the edges of the meadow and the fizzes, schnapps, whistle, and beer begin to take their toll.

A drunk rider slowly slips sideways off his horse. His look is one of confusion and disbelief, then sudden awareness of his inability to recover. Reaching the point of no return, his head and torso swing toward the ground. Clutching a beer in one hand and a cigar in the other, he maintains a death grip on both as he swings earthward. Noiseless as he hits the ground, he lies sprawled just as he hit, not moving for what seems like a very long time. Then a couple of cowboys pick him up and load him in the back of the beer truck. One down and the ride was only an hour old.

"Mount up, boys. It's a trail ride."

Those who still can, mount. The column moves slowly up the hill toward the next clearing, a mile or two along the trail to the next beer stop and a third stop before lunch. The buckaroos spread out across a broad meadow, coveting the shade. Small groups of four to six share a patch of grass, junior members scurrying back and forth with beers to keep senior members, the venerable "viejos," well supplied. The worst possible drink in hot weather is alcohol because it further dehydrates you, and its effect is magnified by dehydration.

"All right, boys, let's turn 'em for home. It's a trail ride."

"Loose horse!" The cry went up as a buckskin quarter horse came bucking and galloping through the line. His saddle had slipped beneath and the stirrups banged his legs as, bucking wildly, he tries to shed the saddle. He was at the end of the meadow and down the trail in an instant, with three cowboys close behind, ropes ready. The last glimpse was of pieces of saddle flying off his back at the end of a noteworthy buck.

The dude who loosened his girth and forgot to tighten it after lunch had paid the price with a broken arm. He lay in the meadow where he had fallen and the paramedic and orthopedic surgeon on the ride were already at work. He'd be back by dinner with a cast and a sheepish look. He would also be appropriately chastised at the kangaroo court on the last night of the ride and his fine would be substantial.

There is no better place to observe the effect of alcohol largely unaffected by social restraint than a trail ride. In fact, hooliganism and barbarous behavior are applauded and venerated. Add unbridled testosterone to the equation and the study in macho intoxication is most educational. It's as if these thirty- to sixty-year-olds had been transported back to their college frat days. It would be amusing and harmless fun if it weren't for the two dozen alcoholics who are given free rein and peer validation for their disease, and the obnoxious behavior those of us who are sober have to endure.

The trail ride evenings are filled with gambling. The man on the far side of the table looks at his cards and pushes in a pile of fifty-dollar bills. He's had too much to drink and he's already lost five thousand dollars, but he won't quit. He just knows his luck will turn; he can will it to change. This doctor is not going to let these uneducated ranchers get the best of him. But the weathered old man two chairs down turns over his cards and shows a king-high straight. With a deadpan expression, he rakes in another thousand dollars of the doctor's cash. At ride's end, he is down ten thousand dollars and has some excuse to make to his (now ex) wife. He never makes the connection between the drinking and the losing; that's why drinks are free at the big casinos. Alcohol has built an empire in Las Vegas. Many of the ride's big losers are as addicted to gambling as they are to alcohol. Their wives dread their return from the ride, the scene that would follow, and the car payment that wouldn't be made that month. And the next year, some won't be on the ride. One is bankrupt; he and the wife are now living with his wife's parents.

After four days, the ride ends and they strike the tent and fold up the craps and poker tables. There are still players sitting at the tables, grizzled beards and eyes like holes burned in a blanket. Some just sit there until the end; others are hoping for the lucky cards, the big pot that would save their marriage and their financial fortunes. And beside them on the table is their umpteenth glass of whiskey.

Why would a sane, sober person subject himself to four days of alcoholic bedlam? At present, I wouldn't. My tolerance for drunks is at an all-time low. Besides, my single weekend ride is three times the distance of the buckaroos' during the entire four-day escapade. But there are other sober people on the ride, three-dozen men whose company, conversation, and character I respect. It would be worth going to spend time with them. I want to disclose that I am a recovering alcoholic, and I hope, by my example, one or two of the buckaroos might see the light and find a way to give up their addiction.

So, I will go back on the trail ride, if I am invited after this book is published. But, I'll watch my back carefully. And you won't find me at the front of that bar.

Dateline: San Jose

PUNCHING GAME ENDS IN
16-YEAR-OLD BOY'S DEATH

A beer-fueled punching game between two teenagers ended in tragedy early Sunday after one of the boys abruptly collapsed and died after being struck with a blow to the chest.

Jacob Salas, 16, was pronounced dead at a Kaiser Permanente hospital in Santa Clara County, authorities said. The boy who struck him, 19-year-old Richard Jimenez, was arrested on suspicion of involuntary manslaughter, according to San Jose police spokesman Sgt. Steve Dixon.

[Author note: Jacob died from either a collapsed lung, a severely bruised myocardium (heart muscle), or a fatal arrhythmia caused by blunt chest trauma.]

28

THE HOLIDAY PARTY

Frank was standing too close, invading my personal space with his paunch and his wineglass.

"You know, Doc, I wanted to be a doctor when I was in high school. I would have made a good one. Blood doesn't bother me at all. I watch the surgery channel all the time."

"What happened that you didn't?" I queried.

"It was too much school. I'd be old before I could make any money." His face was flushed with Cabernet; his eyes were watery.

"It isn't for everybody," I offered, trying to disengage.

"How old were you when you started your practice?"

"Thirty."

"There, you see, Melissa and I had our own home and two kids by that time, and you were just starting out."

It didn't hurt that Melissa's parents had a dozen student rentals that Frank managed and someday would own.

Desperate to escape, I showed Frank my empty punch cup and moved off toward the refreshment table.

For the observant and insightful, holiday parties are a remarkable way to view the effect alcohol has on people—maybe the best. Alcohol's social and psychological lubrication produces behaviors and interactions that are interesting and revealing. The holiday season accentuates emotions. Traditionally a time of friendship and giving, the holidays cause many to struggle with conflicting feelings. There are memories of loved ones lost by death, divorce, or estrangement. Daylight is short and the weather cold. Many find the season depressing and feel disconnected from the holiday revelers around them. A couple of eggnogs laced with brandy helps for a while. Then the depression brought about by the higher dose of alcohol and the dissolution of inhibition creates some very telling scenes.

There is Jim, the rotund physician of Irish descent with the alcoholism to match. He arrives fortified with two scotch and waters and heads straight to the bar. Before long, his eyes are bloodshot and his speech is slurred. He lost his father to alcoholic cirrhosis a year ago, but it hasn't diminished Jim's drinking. His wife tolerates him, but for the last five years she has been squirreling away a good piece of his paycheck. A year from now she'll leave him. Jim will almost die from the loss and the resultant drinking, but an intervention by his brother and a month of rehab will save him. He'll find another wife on the Internet and be back to heavy drinking within a year.

Clarice is married to Howard, the failed trust-fund baby. She appears slightly schizophrenic at parties. She is outwardly warm, friendly, and conversational, but at times her face is sad and distant, unconscious of the fourth glass of wine in her hand. Life didn't turn out as she had planned, but she would never let on. The wine helps her forget the dreams that will never come true.

Dolores stands rigidly at the buffet, drinking short sips of wine as if she were punishing it. She never leaves Harry's side and never stops criticizing his failed investments, lack of dietary willpower, or his family. Nothing escapes her ire as the anger grows with her blood alcohol. Harry accepts it meekly, seemingly in good humor. They have done this dance for twenty-five years.

Then there's Penny. Lipstick a little too red, skirt a little too tight, she arrives at the party already tipsy. When the music starts, she is up and dancing with wild abandon, bumping and grinding through a dozen partners, infuriating wives who have seen her act before and shocking ones who haven't. For a while she'll command the stage, and then the wine will take control and she'll stagger, fall down, or get sick. Later her husband will help her to the car before she passes out on the drive home.

Sally is there as well. Her laugh becomes louder and progressively more annoying. As a single mom with two difficult teenage boys and no help from her ex, she has a hard life. She may be laughing to keep from crying.

These and many other characters often appear at the holiday party. Moderate intoxication unveils secrets of their lives and emotions. If they could see a replay of their actions under the influence, see them as others do, they might gain insight into the problem. They might recognize that the use of alcohol is a symptom of their problem, not the answer to it.

High-functioning alcoholics, the uncommon drunks, are one element of holiday parties. Hard-core alcoholics are more difficult to manage during this season.

My Uncle Jack would have been inducted into the Hall of Fame if one existed for drunks. Pampered and spoiled as a young man, he inherited his father's alcoholic traits. Gifted intellectually, he squandered his college years by drinking heavily. Ironically, we honed our drinking skills at the same university.

Although Uncle Jack had the intellect to achieve anything, the need to drink quenched his desire. He held down a decent job writing technical manuals for an aerospace company for thirty-five years—remarkable considering he was fall-down drunk every day of his career.

Each Christmas Eve, he would show up for my parents' party. It was the only day of the year Jack relinquished his barstool at Alphonse's, his home bar. Arriving fairly sober, by early evening he was drunk and moving through the crowd sharing his intellect and debating skills with the guests. He was very well-read and would argue his point of view even as his tongue thickened through the evening. He was the caricature of a drunk: a worn sport coat open to a white shirt stretched over an ample beer belly, a pointed finger emphasizing his argument. Invariably, accentuating a point, he would accidentally spit on his victim. By evening's end, he had usually insulted several of the guests. I wondered why my parents continued to invite him.

As an adult, I finally asked my mom why. She explained that she had promised her mother that she would look after Jack, including him in holiday celebrations. This was prior to my insight into the nature of high-functioning alcoholism, codependency, and enabling, so I didn't understand. Now I do.

My Uncle Jack died this spring of colon cancer, one of the cancers known to be caused by alcohol. He died alone, penniless, and virtually friendless.

Holiday parties are a fascinating opportunity to see behaviors resultant from the abandonment of normal social inhibitions. For the observant guest, many secrets are revealed. At your next holiday party or wedding, take note of the stereotypes. It may be more painful than reality television. Was there a time when you were among them?

29

LESSONS FROM THE LIBERTY TATTOO CLINIC

The brilliant, rapid-fire yellow flares light the wall behind me. The sound resembles a muffled automatic weapon. The black swastika on Chuck's upper arm disappears four millimeters at a time as the skin frosts white beneath the pulses of laser light. The beam sweeps up and down his tattoo, each pulse removing a tiny bit of hate. Glistening beads of sweat swell on Chuck's forehead as, teeth clenched, he bears the pain. Hunched over, holding his arm, I breathe slow and steady, trying to keep the goggles from fogging over my mask. In several minutes, it is done, the faint red of hemorrhage spreading from the edge of the treated area. Expertly, the wound is covered with aloe vera gel, a gauze pad, and a roll of gauze wrapped securely around the arm to hold it in place.

Chuck is a heavy equipment operator. He is six feet six and a solid 240 pounds, with arms like an NFL lineman. In a prior life, he was the enforcer in a white supremacist prison gang and his appearance is intimidating.

"Doc, I can't thank you enough for what you're doing," he says meekly.

"You're thanking me by staying clean and doing your part to save a few more like you, Chuck."

"Oh, don't worry, Doc. I'm never going down that road again. That road's for losers."

"See you in a couple of months, Chuck."

"You got it, Doc."

This was Chuck's third treatment. At the first, he was stiff and self-conscious, but now he was clearly at ease and friendly. He spent six years in prison for armed robbery as a result of his addiction to methamphetamine and alcohol. His arms were free of the needle marks and scars of some of my heroin addict patients, but they were covered with menacing tattoos.

Slowly, these remnants of his former life were disappearing beneath the flashing beam of our Q-switched neodymium-yttrium-argon-gallium laser (Nd-YAG). The intense laser light, delivered in pulses of a millionth of a second, is absorbed by the small pigment granules that constitute the tattoo. The light is converted to heat and vibration, breaking the granules into small enough pieces for the body to digest. A layer of pigment disappears under the flashing light of the Nd-YAG laser.

Chuck is one of a hundred and fifty patients that I am treating in the Liberty clinic, which offers tattoo removal in return for community service. It is open to anyone with tattoos that are socially offensive or dangerous or that prevent them from obtaining employment or advancing beyond a menial position at their job.

My work at Liberty has been a real education. Three-quarters of my patients are recovering drug and alcohol abusers. Many have been in prison. Most have been as low as human beings can go. Nearly all of them have made a choice to clean up their lives and to regain their self-respect. What a remarkable group of friendly, enthusiastic, grateful, and honest people. It is powerful to learn their stories and to help them rebuild their lives. They all possess a quiet dignity that results from fighting their nearly hopeless battles against alcohol and drugs. And they candidly share their stories with each other and with me. They have taught me a great deal.

The first and most telling fact I learned is that alcohol was the first step in every one of their descents into addiction. For every heroin addict and meth head, the journey started with alcohol.

Second, at the height of their abuse, alcohol remained a mainstay of their addictive behavior. For each it was drug X and *alcohol*. If the drug of choice wasn't available because of supply issues or lack of funds, alcohol was always there, cheap and accessible, to maintain mental oblivion until the next big score. To a person, these recovering addicts don't differentiate between cocaine, liquor, crystal meth, or heroin. It is all the same disease to them. It's not as if they graduated from alcohol to heroin; they just added the heroin to the alcohol.

A review of a few case studies from Liberty Clinic will highlight the effect of alcohol. Chuck, one of my more recent patients, grew up in a blue-collar area of Los Angeles. His father was an alcoholic who beat Chuck and his mother most nights. By the time he was thirteen, Chuck made it a point to be out with his friends at night. He didn't come home until late, when his father had passed out or gone to sleep in an alcoholic stupor. His junior high school friends were all white in a neighborhood with many Hispanics and a few Asians and blacks. In a racial minority, these whites banded together.

Chuck started drinking occasionally when he was ten and regularly when he was thirteen. He joined a white supremacist gang avowed to eliminate all non-whites from their "turf." Its members ranged in age from thirteen to fifty, so buying alcohol was not a problem. Recreational activities included ingesting alcohol, smoking marijuana, taking speed, riding motorcycles, and sharing women.

The gang had graduates in prison and alumni in cemeteries, the victims of gang violence or motorcycling "under the influence." Ironically, I had worked in an emergency room in my residency and met one of them. One of the most horrific injuries I ever dealt with was a senior member of Chuck's gang who, drunk and high on methamphetamine, put his "mama" on the back of his Harley and rode it down the street at 3 AM with no headlights. Lack of headlights was his first mistake; riding the wrong way on a one-way street was his second. He and his girlfriend were hit head-on by a car. The woman was dead at the scene. The rider was folded in half, backward under the car. When he arrived in my emergency room, he was still alive, barely. His head had been crushed on one side so it looked like he had two disparate halves stuck together, and he was in profound shock. I started large IVs and ran in massive amounts of fluid as I rode with him to the trauma center for treatment but, mercifully, he succumbed on the way.

Growing up, Chuck never knew a high school graduate. His compadres either had been arrested or had dropped out to go to work before they graduated. Needing money for drugs and alcohol, he held up a convenience store and was arrested. It wasn't his first. They gave him five to ten and he served six. Life in prison was a racial survival of the fittest. Chuck did what was necessary in order to survive, but along the way he realized that there was no future in his present life. He joined Alcoholics Anonymous and Narcotics Anonymous (NA), and when released, he was fortunate enough to get a job running a backhoe for a contractor who, like him, was a recovering alcoholic and addict. Now he was married with two young children; it was hard to believe Chuck had such a sordid previous life. The tattoos attested to it, but they would soon be gone.

Sally is one of my long-standing laser patients. She has two small remnants of her five tattoos, which will require only a couple more treatments. During her former life as a biker "mama," Sally was an alcoholic and drug addict. While her addiction ran the entire pharmacological gamut from meth to coke and finally to heroin, a period of several years is just a blur in her memory. She did whatever was necessary to get her drugs, often serving as the sexual slave of a dealer. But Sally is adamant that her addiction was never just heroin; it was always alcohol and heroin. She has been clean and sober for fifteen years, and the strength of her commitment to recovery is impressive. Otherwise, she would be dead by now.

Drug addicts live a life of deadly risk. The first and foremost risk is the purity of the drug. Can you imagine buying a substance that you are going to eat or smoke, let alone inject in your veins, from a person that you don't know, don't trust, and are certain would kill you if you missed a payment? This is the addict's world. How do you know the crystal meth is pure? What is it cut with? How strong is the heroin? One of the more common scenarios in heroin addiction is death from overdose, as every batch is of a different potency. The same dose you shot up last time may kill you this time, or it may have little or no effect. One of the heroin ODs I treated while running the overdose ward at LA County-USC Hospital was brought up as a "red blanket." He was comatose, was barely breathing, and had pinpoint pupils, a sure sign of heroin intoxication. He was very well-dressed and there was something strikingly familiar about him. As I drew up the Narcan (the antidote to heroin), I studied his face. Then it hit me. He was an actor, star of my favorite TV western. I gave him the Narcan, and within several minutes he was wide-awake, embarrassed, and ashamed. He had been attending a party at another celebrity's home in the Malibu Colony. Everyone had been drinking pretty heavily when a close female friend suggested they try some heroin. He had tried it several times before with pleasant results and, wanting to please her, said yes. She injected him and that's the last he remembered until he awakened, looking up at a fresh-faced intern in a white jacket. If the heroin had been a little more potent, he would have died of respiratory arrest. He was lucky that someone was aware enough to call 911, that the paramedics responded so quickly, and that the emergency medical system worked so well. For most addicts, that would not have been the case. Liberty Program's recovering addicts have lost a lot of friends to overdoses.

There is an unusual risk with intravenous heroin use: sudden death. It's not an overdose and it's not an allergic reaction. It's some kind of toxicity that just kills instantly. Addicts are found with needles still in their arms, cold and stiff.

Additionally there are the risks of infection, such as hepatitis B and C, HIV, and the common bacterial infections like staph and strep. Add to that the sexually transmitted infections that occur with the lifestyle and behaviors of addicts, and it becomes clear that drug use incurs monumental risk.

What does this have to do with alcohol? Quite a bit. First, all my recovering addict friends started with alcohol, and alcohol was always an integral part of their addiction. Second, alcohol impairs judgment and promotes risky behaviors including use of other drugs and dangerous sexual habits. My chagrined TV western star clearly stated they had all been drinking heavily at the party before the heroin came out.

People die of alcohol addiction much more frequently than they do of heroin addiction. It may be from an auto accident while driving drunk, an alcoholic committing suicide after abandoning all hope, a blow to the head in a drunken brawl, or perhaps from acute or chronic alcohol poisoning. Whatever the scenario, the cause is constant: that two-carbon ethanol so enthusiastically promoted by the advertising media and accepted everywhere in polite society.

Perhaps it's time for a reevaluation.

DAVID BREWER

He looked guilty as charged. He sat on the exam table looking not like a patient but like a serial killer just apprehended. His dark eyes looked tired and sad. Thirty years old, he had gone to school with my daughter. He was strikingly handsome but had the look of a homeless person. He had a reputation a decade ago for drinking and fighting. The beads of sweat on his forehead, the sour smell of last night's beer on his breath, the clammy handshake, and the fine tremor in his fingers told me his alcohol and drug addiction had progressed since I last saw him. I suspected he was in heroin withdrawal. He had been twenty minutes late for his appointment, but with premalignant moles and with the real risk that he will have a deadly melanoma in the future, I saw him anyway. I tried to be friendly but his look was vacant and he responded in mono-syllables. No, he wasn't working. Yes, he was still living in town.

My sense was of a soul in purgatory. If only I could say something, do something, to give him hope. I felt helpless. I finished my exam and left the room as he dropped his head and returned to his personal hell.

30

WHEN YOUR LUCK RUNS OUT: DUI

It's half past eleven. There's not much traffic on the freeway as you head home from a party. Sally is silent in the seat beside you. You're thinking about Fred's potential stock deal, not really paying attention to your driving.

Suddenly, there are flashing red lights in your rearview mirror and you are gripped with fear. You've been drinking, like the hundred other nights over the years when you haven't been stopped, when you went home slightly tipsy but confident that you could still drive well enough not to attract attention.

You pull to the side of the road, fighting an overwhelming panic. After all these years that you've gotten away with it, your charmed life with drinking and driving is about to come to an end.

The patrolman has shined his auxiliary spot into the back of your car and the light is blinding. A flashlight approaches from the rear and comes to a stop by your window. You lower it and the officer's face is six inches from yours. He's sniffing the air in the car and your breath.

"What's the matter, officer?" you say calmly, trying to fight back the fear.

"Good evening. May I see your driver's license, please?"

"Yes, sir. What's the matter, officer?" He's watching you very carefully as you get out your wallet, evaluating your coordination. You open the wallet and hand it to him with the license still in its plastic holder.

"Take it out, please. Just the license." Officer Margaroli is a thirty-year veteran of the Highway Patrol and he's seen it all. Many times he's had drivers hand him the open wallet and in the plastic liner facing the license is a fifty- or hundred-dollar bill.

Fighting panic, you slowly peel the license from its plastic cover and hand it to the officer. You won't see it again for six months, if then.

"Is there a problem, officer?"

He carefully looks at the license and then at you. "You were having a little difficulty maintaining your lane, Mr. Jones. Have you been drinking tonight?" Officer Margaroli calls it "driving by the numbers": the vehicle slowly drifts out of the lane, there is an abrupt correction, then it drifts again, then a correction, and so on.

"Yes sir. We were at a dinner party, but I only had two glasses of wine all evening," you lie. You had two beers before dinner, three glasses of wine with dinner, and a glass of port with dessert: nine and a half ounces of alcohol.

Margaroli can smell the alcohol off-gassing from your lungs. He's pretty sure you are over the legal limit for driving.

"Mr. Jones, I'd like to do a simple test. Don't move your head, just your eyes. Follow my fingers." The officer looks straight at you. He extends one finger in front of your nose vertically and you focus on it. Then he moves it out to the side and you follow his finger with your eyes, keeping your head still. The officer is intent. He is looking for nystagmus, an involuntary horizontal twitching of the eyes that is characteristic of intoxication. It is caused by a disparity in strength of the medial and lateral rectus, those muscles controlling the horizontal movement of the eye, and it can be a very good indication of the level of intoxication. The sooner it appears, as the subject looks outward, the drunker the subject is. Your nystagmus begins about halfway across the range of motion: moderate intoxication.

"Mr. Jones, do you know what nystagmus is?"

"No."

"You don't have hereditary or idiopathic nystagmus?"

"No."

"I am going to have to do some additional tests. Would you get out of the car, please? Leave your lights on."

You get out of the car and walk behind him to the front where the headlights illumine a large area for his field sobriety tests.

"Just stand right here." He places you in front of the car, your back to it, facing him.

"Now, stand up straight, put your arms down to your sides, and pick up your left foot. Keep it up for ten seconds."

You follow his directions and lift your left foot. You immediately sway to the right, overcorrect to the left, overcorrect again, and have to put your left foot down. The officer is doing the same exercise, beginning to count. He only gets to four when your foot again hits the pavement.

"Let's try the right."

Again, you square yourself and lift your right foot. This time your torso swings in a big circle and it widens until your right foot finally hits the ground again, just short of your falling down. The officer counted to eight.

"Okay, Mr. Jones, let's try another." Officer Margaroli's suspicions are being confirmed. "Stand up straight, at attention, heels together, arms out, look up at the stars, then close your eyes." The officer demonstrates.

Completely humiliated, you comply. You are fine until you look up and then the torso again begins to circle and you know you are going to fall. You straighten your head and regain your balance. You're zero for four.

"Let's try one more, shall we?" The officer hands you a pen and a pad of paper. "Write the alphabet for me. Take your time. Make sure you get it right."

Totally flustered, you slowly and carefully write the alphabet on his small scratch pad and hand it back to him. At least that's one you can't miss.

He looks it over. "You left out *U* and *V*," he reports. "I am going to ask you to breathe into our Preliminary Alcohol Screening Device. You don't have to do this since it is just a field sobriety test, but if I arrest you for driving under the influence, you must submit to and complete a formal blood alcohol test. Either a blood or breath sample will be taken."(You, as the suspected intoxicated motorist, can no longer refuse all testing. The courts have decided that since driving is a privilege and not a right, there are implied responsibilities that accompany that privilege, one of which is to submit to alcohol testing on demand.)

The officer holds a small black plastic box in front of your mouth. It has a straw-like device extending horizontally out of the top.

"Take a deep breath and blow into this, Mr. Jones."

You comply and blow hard into the device. You hear a whistle like a New Year's Eve party favor. The officer then pushes a button on the side of the box and you hear a loud "click." He examines it carefully with his flashlight.

"Mr. Jones, I am afraid I am going to have to arrest you for driving under the influence of alcohol."

You are numb. All your worst fears are finally realized. He takes out a pair of handcuffs and submissively you extend both wrists.

"Behind your back, please." He is kind. He acts as if he truly feels sorry for you. He locks the handcuffs on your wrists behind your back and guides you over to the back door of the patrol car. You slip in and the door closes behind you.

The officer talks to Sally and determines she is not under the influence (it's very important not to arrest one DUI and let another drive away). He tells her to drive your car home and wait for a call from you. If there are no hitches, it will be four to six hours.

You hear him radio in something to dispatch. "This is unit…. Bringing in suspect Jones for booking on 23152 A and B." It's the first time you've heard those numbers, but it won't be the last.

There is silence all the way to county jail, interrupted at intervals by the terse staccato of radio communication from the dispatcher. In the brightly lit parking lot, Officer Margaroli opens the door and assists you out, then walks you through the double glass doors of the entryway and into the booking unit of the jail.

Your handcuffs are removed. Officer Margaroli explains that you have to blow again into another Breathalyzer. This one is a more technologically sophisticated instrument called an "intoxicimeter." The test you took at the roadside was a preliminary determination, enough to proceed with an arrest. The intoxicimeter is a device with high scientific accuracy, the test results of which are admissible in court. It is calibrated weekly.

You blow into the straw-like mouthpiece, and after a few seconds, the digital readout shows the blood level: 0.16 percent, twice the legal limit.

Officer Margaroli turns you over to the county booking officer and returns to his patrol. You will not see him again unless your case goes to trial and he is called as a witness.

The uniformed booking agent gives you a large manila envelope and asks you to put your wallet, jewelry, and all valuables in it. No jewelry is allowed in the jail. Even your wedding ring goes into the envelope. He asks you a number of questions and fills out two long forms. You have a blinding headache now, and the glare of the lights in the booking area is painfully bright. You are asked about any identifying marks, tattoos, scars, birthmarks, missing digits. You are searched completely by a male deputy and then you are fingerprinted: the thumb and all the fingers of your right hand.

Then, you are led into a holding cell, a large glass enclosure adjacent to the booking area. There are chairs and a phone. You may make all the local calls you wish. The sheriff's staff will run a computer search on you in the next few hours, and if you have no outstanding warrants or a prior record, you will be released on your own recognizance after four hours.

You call Sally, ashamed and humiliated. You are all right, and you will call her again when they release you.

Four hours seems like an eternity. By the time you are finally released, you call your wife, and she picks you up, it is 5 AM. They return the manila envelope with all your valuables. You have a pink piece of paper, which is your temporary driver's license, and a court date to appear for a preliminary hearing.

There is silence in the car all the way home. Sally has never criticized or complained about your drinking. She doesn't drink every day like you do, but at parties she drinks nearly as much as you do, and until tonight she never had to worry about driving home because you were seemingly sober enough to get home without difficulty.

All that has now changed. You are a drunk driver.

One of the longest nights of your life has finally ended, but the nightmare is just beginning.

The next day, Sunday, you call an old and trusted friend who is an attorney. He doesn't do criminal defense or drunk driving, but he knows the legal community and he knows the process you'll follow. You meet at his house and spend an hour learning what you need to do and how it's going to work for the next few months. First, you need a lawyer. Dave knows a couple of good ones who are experienced. You will hire one and he will guide you through the legal maze.

First of all, your driver's license will be sent to the DMV and you will not see it again until your suspension is over. You can drive on your temporary license until your trial, but if you are convicted, your license will be automatically suspended for six months. Since it is your first offense, you may obtain permission to drive to and from work.

You will have a preliminary hearing in the next several weeks to set a court date for trial. Your lawyer can appear for you. Then he will examine the evidence and try to employ legal sleight of hand to get you off or to plead you to a lesser charge than "driving under the influence."

The system has left several gaping loopholes that occasionally prove very helpful in getting a client a reduced charge and sentence. But the process is fraught with anxiety for the charged and can be quite costly.

Six months of your life are turned upside down. Your attorney is good, but the case against you is pretty tight. Attorneys often try to attack the rationale for the officer's stopping the suspect, claiming that there was not sufficient "probable cause" and the officer was just "fishing." In your case, you were observed driving erratically. Strike one.

You failed the field sobriety tests. Strike two.

You blew a 0.161 percent blood alcohol on the intoxicimeter at the jail, an instrument that was calibrated the day prior and whose accuracy is unquestioned by the court. Strike three.

Your attorney negotiates with the district attorney handling your case. Since this was your first offense and you have a completely clean driving record without even a speeding ticket in the last ten years, he bargains to reduce the charge to a misdemeanor called a "wet reckless": reckless driving with an elevated blood alcohol. It's just a legal game but it makes a huge difference. A "wet reckless" does not appear on your permanent driving record as drunk driving, the fine is not as steep, you don't lose your driver's license, and you are not required to go to Alcohol School, which is the alcohol equivalent of Traffic Safety School.

But it costs you $5,000 for the attorney, $500 more in yearly insurance premiums, and humiliation. You live in a small town, so everyone knows you were busted.

Maybe it's the impetus you need to finally recognize that you have a problem with alcohol, that you are becoming an alcoholic. Or perhaps after reading and imagining this mortifying process, you don't need to experience it firsthand. Before you have to endure the emotional trauma, you can admit there is a growing problem and get help. Before you end up as one of the twenty-five thousand traffic fatalities caused by alcohol each year. Before you are responsible for killing or seriously injuring an innocent person, even perhaps a child, and living the rest of your life with that guilt. You don't have to wait for the flashing lights in your rearview mirror. Seek help now.

NO HELP AT THE JAIL

The hole in Luke's forehead was quarter-sized but the cancer was gone. Fortunately, it had not gone to the bone. Still it would be a challenge to close the defect. Luke is a recovering alcoholic and a drug and alcohol therapist with the county.

"So I am told that they don't have any drug and alcohol therapists at the jail anymore."

"Yeah. Haven't had for nearly two years."

"Why?"

"Sheriff didn't want to pay for them. Budget cuts and all that."

"But that seems like such a critical place to be. Somebody just gets busted, that's when you're the most likely to reach them."

"Yeah, you're right. But we're at the bottom of the food chain when it comes to funding and priorities."

"Is it because the perception is that alcohol rehab isn't very effective?"

"Partly, but I think there's something else."

"What?"

"I think it hits a little close to home."

"You mean a lot of decision makers in county government and law enforcement have their own issues with it?"

"You didn't hear me say that. But maybe so."

Upwards of 60 percent of inmates in California prisons have a history of drug and alcohol abuse. More than 50 percent of homicides, vehicular deaths, and child and spousal abuse involve alcohol. Effective alcohol treatment should be the first weapon in the crime prevention arsenal. Why is it the last?

Luke's forehead closed nicely. Alcoholism is a cancer in our society that is not as readily removed as Luke's cancer. We would have a higher success rate if we had the political will to make it happen.

31

OBSERVATIONS OF A HIGHWAY PATROL OFFICER

Officer Chuck Margaroli (Badge #8533), whom I interviewed for the previous chapter, has worked for the California Highway Patrol for thirty years. He has arrested countless drunk drivers and seen innumerable auto accidents with injuries and fatalities caused by intoxicated drivers.

I asked him candidly what he'd like to see change about our drunk-driving laws or the way they are enforced. He responded that the decreased tolerance for the drunk driver, both by the public and by law enforcement, is a positive change that's long overdue. And yet, those who are outraged by a driver with a blood alcohol of 0.24 percent who drives the wrong direction on the freeway and kills a mother and her two young children in a head-on collision will drive home from a party with a blood alcohol of 0.12 percent without a second thought. It's always someone else who has the drinking problem. Chuck would like to see people wake up that it's "their problem, too."

Chuck has noticed a significant increase in drunk driving since the terrorist attacks of 9/11. He attributes it to general anxiety in the community about the future safety of our country and our world.

The law enforcement community's focus on holiday drinking has decreased drunk driving on the holidays themselves, through a heightened public awareness of consequences and the increased use of designated drivers. But it's not just Thanksgiving, Christmas, and New Year's that are the problem: It's the entire holiday season. Drunken driving arrests and accidents increase throughout, beginning at Thanksgiving and continuing through New Year's. He attributes holiday parties for fueling the problem.

Officer Margaroli is pleased with the stringent laws punishing drunk drivers, notably the enhanced penalties for driving under the influence with a child (under fourteen) in the vehicle, the enhanced penalties for having a blood alcohol in excess of 0.20 percent, and the mandatory jail term for a fourth offense. But, he is frustrated with the judicial system's enforcement of the laws, particularly judges who throw out solid cases on legal technicalities. They have cast doubt repeatedly on his or other officers' judgment and have implied that the officer was overzealous in his pursuit of a particular case or that he may have "bent" the truth in order to establish certain evidence. For example, on one occasion, Officer Margaroli and his partner were parked at a stop sign on the outskirts of one of the South County beach cities. A lady returning home after an afternoon of golf and an evening of drinking at the nearby country club literally skidded through the stop sign and intersection in front of them. They stopped her for running the stop sign. They observed somewhat intoxicated behavior while interviewing her. She failed field sobriety tests and "blew" a 0.18 percent blood alcohol on the preliminary alcohol screening (PAS) device. Chuck and his partner arrested her. At the jail she blew a 0.16 percent alcohol on the more accurate and court-admissible intoxicimeter.

This case of intoxication while driving was dismissed. The defendant's attorney submitted a weather report stating there was dense fog that night. He insisted that the officers could not possibly have observed the defendant skidding through the stop sign, that they did not have "probable cause" to stop her. He filed a motion to suppress all the evidence of her intoxication that was gleaned subsequent to her being stopped.

Officer Margaroli explained that the fog was patchy and that they had a clear view of the intersection, but the judge threw the case out on the attorney's motion.

That needs to stop.

Officer Margaroli also would like to see a relatively new defense strategy called the "rising blood alcohol" defense disallowed. Say, for instance, a driver is stopped, is judged to show signs of intoxication, and blows a 0.08 percent blood alcohol. At the jail, he blows a 0.10 percent blood alcohol and is booked for drunk driving. The attorneys will argue that the defendant had a drink just before the arrest and that the alcohol was still being assimilated. Since at the time it was checked it was barely the legal limit for intoxication, it was in fact lower than that when the defendant was stopped. Therefore, the defendant was not legally intoxicated.

Our veteran patrolman vigorously applauds the zero-tolerance policy for minors. Under the present laws, anyone under twenty-one may have no alcohol in their blood. If they do, it is an automatic two-year suspension of their driver's license. Since teen drinking is a persistent and growing problem, it doesn't keep young people from drinking, but it has gone a long way toward keeping them off the road when they have been drinking.

When I asked him to cite the drunk-driving case that he remembered most vividly, he recounted a story of a local dentist who had been drinking at a seaside bar. Driving home at a high rate of speed, he lost control of his vehicle on a tight turn called "Screech Owl Curve," well-known for the many accidents that have occurred there. His car crossed the center divider and hit an oncoming compact car. The dentist was driving a large Mercedes, and although it was nearly totaled, he was unhurt. Miraculously, the driver of the compact was not killed, but he sustained massive injuries including two broken legs, a dislocated shoulder, and extensive facial fractures and lacerations.

The dentist had a blood alcohol in excess of 0.20 percent. He pleaded "no contest" to driving under the influence. By doing this, he is not admitting guilt in a civil suit which could follow the criminal action of his drunk-driving trial. The victim spent years enduring reconstructive surgery and rehabilitating his extensive orthopedic injuries. He will never return to his "pre-accident" state and will carry the scars and pains of his injuries for the remainder of his life. The dentist, virtually unscathed, was sentenced to a six-month license suspension and attendance at Alcohol School, in addition to his automobile insurance premiums rising $2,000 a year.

What's wrong with this picture?

Recently, a police dispatcher from our local university was killed by a drunk driver. The dispatcher was stopped at a signal on Highway One when a drunk driver, oblivious to the stopped vehicle, slammed into the back of her car. The force of the impact severed the spine of the stationary driver and she died of her massive injuries after a week in the intensive care unit of a local hospital. The drunk driver had a blood alcohol of 0.17 percent and this was his *sixth offense* for drunk driving. When I asked the patrolman how a five-time offender was allowed back on the road, he simply answered, "We don't allow him. He was driving on a revoked license."

The driver was tried for vehicular manslaughter and convicted. The original sentence was seven years, which was later increased to eleven on the special circumstances of repeat offenses. How can we get these repeat offenders off the road? If they disregard the law and drive drunk on suspended and revoked licenses, perhaps they need to be incarcerated to protect the population against their public menace.

After thirty years on the job, Officer Margaroli knows when to expect a lot of drunks on the road. Sunny weekends are always bad. The beer starts flowing after noon and by mid-to-late afternoon, when the cowboys are all heading home, most of them have a snoot full. Given that a lot of drinking starts in the mid-to-late afternoon and continues on into the evening, the peak times for drunk drivers is 5 PM to 11 PM on the weekends. Another significant time period is just after 2 AM when the bars close.

Asked which drunk drivers are the most difficult to handle, the officer is automatic in his response: It's the women. They are all sweetness and light when first stopped, certain that they can flirt their way out of an arrest. When it is apparent that arrest is inevitable, they turn into witches, or worse. Officer Margaroli reports that the most vile language he has ever heard came from the mouth of that same woman who five minutes before was the picture of decorum.

Asked what was the highest blood alcohol he has ever seen in his long career, he relates a story of an arrest he made within the last decade. He was making a traffic stop for a speeding driver. Pulled to the side of the road with the previously speeding vehicle, the officer noticed a car pull up behind him. A man got out and staggered toward him. Slurring his words, the man asked for directions to a location several miles down the road. After a brief interview and failed field sobriety tests, the man blew into the PAS apparatus. The patrolman was astounded to see the results: 0.36 percent. Most with a blood alcohol at that level would be barely conscious, certainly not upright and walking. Chuck arrested the man and took him to jail, but he could not be prosecuted for drunk driving because he was not observed driving, only drunk in public, a much less serious offense.

Officer Margaroli has some sage advice for anyone who would drink and drive: "Don't do it." You may escape notice for years, but the slightest error may send a ton and a half of steel careening off the highway or into another vehicle and you may be charged with murder or at least vehicular manslaughter. Imagine living with the guilt of injuring or killing someone. Have someone else, someone sober, drive you home before you see those flashing red lights in your rearview mirror and your life changes forever.

32

ENABLING

"The mystery masked man was smart,
He got himself a Tonto.
Tonto did the dirty work for free."

—*Lyle Lovett*

Nancy is one of the nicest people you would ever want to meet. Mid-sixties and athletic-looking, Nancy has run a number of fifty-kilometer and fifty-mile ultra-marathons, winning her age group on several occasions and setting records along the way. Kind, soft-spoken, an excellent cook, and a hard worker, Nancy is a pleasure to be around.

So why does this remarkable woman choose to live with hopeless alcoholics?

She lost her first husband to alcoholism. By all accounts, Ron was abusive, yet she remained with him. Totally lost in his addiction, Ron was sitting at a bar one evening with Nancy at his side, when suddenly he fell backward onto the floor: dead. The cumulative effect of thirty years of hard drinking combined to scar his liver and weaken his heart. Insidiously, fluid began to back up in his lungs from a heart poisoned by alcohol. The cough that had worsened in the preceding week wasn't a virus. It was fluid filling the alveoli, the air sacs, throughout his lungs. It's kind of like drowning, from the inside. When nearly half the lungs are flooded, there is not enough surface area to absorb oxygen. The blood oxygen plummets, and at some critical level the myocardium or heart muscle, already weakened from the toxic effect of high blood alcohol, suddenly misfires and goes into a fatal ventricular fibrillation. Ron was dead before he hit the floor.

Within eighteen months, Nancy had met and married Larry, another alcoholic. Larry was less abusive, although when he drank he could be incredibly demeaning. Larry functioned at a remarkably high level. He was employed by a utility company for thirty years, trained countless hours on a bicycle, and had bought property and was building a beautiful house in the foothills of the north county. But, he was drunk every day.

What is it about a person like Nancy that would make her enter into another relationship with an alcoholic? Nancy drinks, but not every day. I've never seen her drunk. She is always sober enough to drive Larry home from a barbecue. So why does she do it?

Nancy is codependent. There is something about the relationship that she needs or wants or she wouldn't stay in it. What does she want?

In my experience, there are three types of people who choose to stay in relationships like Nancy's. The first is the classic enabler, a person who facilitates the life and activities of the alcoholic because she needs him to complete her identity. The concept is a little difficult to grasp but is best explained by the Greek myth of Narcissus and Echo. Narcissus was a lesser god who was quite handsome and enjoyed admiring himself, to the exclusion of anyone around him. Echo, a wood nymph, was madly in love with Narcissus, but she had been cursed by the goddess Hera for being too talkative. She could only speak in response to someone conversing with her. Echo's opportunity to speak with Narcissus soon occurred, but he spurned her. As a result, the goddess Nemesis caused Narcissus to fall hopelessly in love with his reflection in a pool of water. Thus the myth describes a critical symbiosis between a self-absorbed person oblivious to those around him and another who has no voice, or identity, except as an echo or extension of the first.

Narcissus, a person so self-involved that he is concerned only with himself and his own welfare, parallels closely the alcoholic. Echo is the person with low self-esteem who does not feel she is a complete personality without the alcoholic. Echo does not feel she exists without the dominant selfish personality of Narcissus. Echo has a huge stake in ensuring that Narcissus is able to function because she is dependent on him for her survival. So, even though Narcissus is drunk most of the time, Echo enables him to pursue his alcoholism by handling the everyday details of his life.

So we have Echo doing all she can to enable Narcissus to function better, even though he is a hopeless drunk. That's Nancy. She is the prototype enabler. She has accepted Larry's drinking and makes allowances for it in her life. In return for her tacit acceptance, she gets the security of a nice house, a pension, a body to interact with (although frequently drunk), and a fair amount of control and decision making in the relationship.

It seems a contradiction that Nancy would have any control in the relationship. She is the quiet one, always in the background, allowing Larry to be loud, drunk, and apparently dominant. But because Larry is frequently drunk, he abdicates much of the decision making in the relationship. He yields much of the power by virtue of the fact that he isn't functioning rationally a portion of the time. Additionally, Larry experiences some guilt, although never articulated, giving Nancy the upper hand.

As an enabler, Nancy claims most of the power and shoulders only half the responsibility. She enjoys the creature comforts and the companionship. For her, it is not such a bad deal.

When you analyze the dynamics of the alcoholic, codependent relationship, it is much easier to understand why someone would remain. In the end, however, it all unravels, like Nancy's first marriage did when Ron died. Odds are that alcohol will kill her second husband as well.

The second personality type that coexists with the alcoholic is a very controlling person who uses the alcohol to usurp the power in the relationship. Margaret was like that. She came from substantial wealth and she was used to having her own way. She married Phil, a genuine war hero, after he was discharged in 1945. As they raised their family in the San Joaquin Valley, Phil's drinking progressively worsened. Margaret did nothing to intervene. On the contrary, she used the fact that he was drunk much of the time to become the dominant force in the family and the relationship. Phil abdicated his role as head of the household, which she gladly assumed. This continued until they retired to the Central Coast. Phil got a couple of DUIs and the court mandated he go to AA. He got sober twice, but he relapsed both times. Margaret was secretly happy because his sobriety threatened the balance of power in the relationship. She liked him hopeless and dependent on her. She had not anticipated the possibility, however, that a defeated Phil would commit suicide and end the relationship for good. Amazingly, within a year, Margaret had met and married another alcoholic and had set up a new fiefdom with him.

The last type of enabler is the individual who is in total denial of the alcoholic's problem. Betty is like that. Her twenty-five-year-old son, Eric, has had three DUIs in the last year. He has been fired from his job and the county put his three-year-old son in a foster home. He got another DUI last week. Betty was outraged.

"It wasn't fair. He wasn't really drunk. He'd just had a couple of beers and he was driving home, but the registration on his car had expired and he was pulled over."

I asked what his blood alcohol was.

"He blew a 0.12 percent, but that's not really very high. He'd just had a couple of beers."

Betty doesn't get it. She is blind to the truth that Eric is an alcoholic and that he can't drink at all, not even a couple of beers! By failing to acknowledge his problem, she is enabling his alcoholism. Betty tries to shield her son from the natural consequences of his alcoholic behavior, which is simply postponing the inevitable.

Another example of enabling is demonstrated by Bob and JoAnn Williams. Aging seniors, their daughter, Sally, is a hopeless alcoholic. When her husband left and took the kids after eight dismal, drunken years of marriage, Sally's parents bought her a condo. They give her an allowance so she can survive, and drink, without having to worry about work. Now in their eighties, they are arranging a trust to provide for Sally after their deaths. They are resigned to the fact that Sally is a chronic alcoholic and have made it possible for her to continue her alcoholism without adverse consequences after they are gone. Most would see the flawed logic, but the Williams think they are doing the right thing.

Denial and enabling come in many forms. Recently, we had a drunken riot in our small college town. Revelers, supposedly celebrating Mardi Gras, destroyed cars and street signs and attacked the police when they arrived to disperse the mob. Over a hundred young people were arrested. One was a nineteen-year-old, videotaped by the police lighting a large explosive device, which his friend then threw at the police. Fortunately, the bomb exploded without hitting the officers, but many had ear injuries from the blast.

The young man was arrested and placed in the county jail. Within twenty-four hours, his father, a wealthy Silicone Valley attorney, had written a $500,000 check to bail him out. It was the largest check ever written for bail in our county. The father, when reached for comment, explained that he didn't want his son to have the negative and frightening experience of spending any more time in jail.

The son, who might have learned a better lesson from spending a few more days in county jail, now knows that his father can and will literally bail him out when he gets drunk and commits criminal acts.

A tragic mistake is repeated countless times every day. Yet when there are no negative consequences, there is no learning. It implies that the drunkenness is acceptable behavior, for which individuals and society simply need to provide and adjust.

Tell that to the husband who lost his wife and child in a head-on collision with a drunk; to the police sergeant who has no hearing in his left ear; to the young woman raped at a fraternity party.

They may have a different view.

33

ARE YOU OR IS SOMEONE YOU LOVE AN ALCOHOLIC? HOW TO TELL AND WHAT TO DO

It's time to get personal. Most likely, you are reading this book because of your interest in alcoholism from an intimate perspective. Perhaps you suspect that you are living with an alcoholic, or maybe you know that you have a problem but don't know what to do. Good for you and for having the courage to look for help! The good news is that 30 percent of alcoholics stay sober forever. But, in order to do so, you or your loved one has to realize and accept that there is a problem and make the commitment to change.

Are you an alcoholic? You already know, whether or not you will admit it. It's a very difficult thing to say. That's why the AA route may not, initially, be for everyone. It wasn't for me. To stand up in front of a group of people and say, "My name's Jeff and I'm an alcoholic" was something I was not able to do at first. Was it pride? No. It was shame. I was raised in an environment that equated actions with value. If you did something bad, you were a bad person. My behavior and actions growing up were controlled and shaped by shame and guilt. It has taken decades of reading, prayer, and personal growth to come to the awareness that good people can do bad things and still remain good people. We are all human and at times subject to human weakness. We are individually and collectively capable of messing up, and we do so quite regularly. It doesn't change our essential goodness, but it does require that we acknowledge our actions, feel sincerely sorry for them, and work to avoid similar mistakes in the future. We must believe in forgiveness for ourselves and we need to practice it with others. Truly forgiven, we are free from the burden of our mistakes and from the shame and guilt that attend them. This simple awareness has been so liberating that it has changed my life. But, it didn't change me enough in the beginning to make me want to proclaim my sins in front of a group of strangers. I had to find another way. This may be true as well for you or your loved one.

Back to the question. Are you an alcoholic? Although you already know, often it is on a subconscious level. You may not be aware yet on a conscious level. You may need some prodding.

Let's start with the conventional criteria. Answer yes or no to the following:

Do you drink every day?

Consuming alcohol every day produces brain chemical changes that create a physiological addiction. Even if you don't feel addicted or notice a psychological addiction, there are changes in your body chemistry that now require the presence of alcohol and, with time, will cause other adverse chemical changes when alcohol is withdrawn. When exposed to alcohol, some of the neurotransmitters in the brain's nerve cells rapidly acquire the "need" for alcohol to function, and they malfunction when it is withdrawn. Of course, the severe form of this is delirium tremens, but even with continuous moderate alcohol consumption there are subtle unpleasant biochemical and physiological changes when alcohol is withdrawn. Perhaps it is just an uneasiness or a mild depression when you skip a day of drinking. So consciously or not, you learn not to miss a day. You're addicted.

Have you lost a job because of drinking?

This is one of the classic definitions of alcoholism and one of the most valid for the obvious abuser. But short of being terminated, there are more subtle signs in the workplace of an excessive fondness for drink that are suggestive of a growing problem. Maybe it's missing work or chronic tardiness because you were hungover from a night of drinking. Perhaps it is poor job performance, anger, or quarrelsome behavior brought on by the drinking. These signs are clearly identifiable and few would argue they are the results of an alcohol problem. But for every drinker who loses his job or struggles on with barely tolerable evaluations because of these obvious problems, there are ten workplace high-functioning alcoholics who chronically underperform at work because of alcohol. They accomplish little after noon because of their two-drink lunches causing drowsiness during the second half of the day. They get no take-home work done because they are worthless once they start drinking in the evening.

In the liberated days of the sixties when the baby boomers experimented with drugs, much was made of the "amotivational syndrome" caused by chronic marijuana use. The old aphorism "going to pot" was coined a half century before sophisticated psychological tests defined the problem. Alcohol has the same effect on many people, creating a personal inertia that slows their careers, financial growth, and personal development. When one has a blood alcohol of 0.1 percent every night, it's hard to get much done.

Have you ended a relationship because of drinking?

Divorce or its equivalent is one of the most common occurrences in an alcoholic's life. The alcoholic creates so many impassable roadblocks in the relationship that it turns into a nightmare for the nonalcoholic partner. Whether it is economic insecurity from being fired for drinking on the job, verbal or physical abuse, social embarrassment, or just the growing realization that alcohol is more important than the relationship, the nonalcoholic spouse or partner endures a series of hellish experiences before finally giving up. Oftentimes, the resultant breakup causes the alcoholic to spin further out of control.

But just as there are untold thousands of workplace alcoholics whose behavior never reaches the threshold for termination, there are millions of men and women who struggle in silence with partners who are chronically intoxicated, rude, and deprecating and who make the lives of their significant others barely tolerable. At a party Molly averts her eyes when Larry spills his wine or makes a rude remark. But she is always there to drive him home, enabling him to continue his alcoholism. Molly's insecurity keeps her there. A relationship with a drunk is better than no relationship at all.

Does this sound familiar? Does alcohol dominate your relationship?

Have you been arrested for drunk driving?

For many alcoholics, this is the wake-up call that they have lost touch with the seriousness of their drinking. It is public humiliation and is often the jolt they need to realize that their life is in a downward spiral. Many seek help and find it. Others, still deep in denial, just curse their bad luck at getting caught, hire an attorney who is expert at damage control, and go on with their intoxicated lives. Alcoholics are conditioned to blame their problems on other people or on fate. Rarely do they take responsibility.

Wisely, many states require the person cited for DUI to take a class or enroll in an alcohol rehab program. Another excellent idea would be to sentence the convicted DUI to forty hours of volunteer work at the local alcohol detox unit.

For many early-stage alcoholics, a close-up look at where they are heading is shocking enough to bring about long-term change. Drunk drivers are frequently sentenced to hours of community service, but too often they can pick and choose their assignment and there is no learning or behavior modification that results. I volunteer with the local state park maintaining trails. At a recent work project we had two convicted DUIs fulfilling their community service requirement. One was so hungover that he was worthless; the other drove to the 8 AM project reeking of booze. There was no real supervision or any negative consequences for continued alcoholic behavior.

For every convicted drunk driver, there are a multitude of social drinkers who regularly drive home from parties with blood alcohol levels greater than 0.08 percent, the legal limit in most states. Are you one of them? The fact that we try to get away with it is good evidence that alcohol impairs judgment. Driving under the influence also erodes morality: we know that it is wrong but do it anyway. We are on the slippery slope of alcoholism, explaining away verbal or physical abuse or adultery, behaviors we disparage when sober. It is such a subtle line that we don't realize we have crossed it. And alcohol facilitated our crossing.

Are you restless and ill at ease when not drinking?

The anxiety many alcoholics experience when sober is a combination of feeling socially ill at ease without some alcohol in their bloodstream and actual physiological withdrawal caused by malfunctioning neurons in the brain that have become dependent on the presence of alcohol to work correctly. The alcoholic enters a social gathering looking for the bar, and once it is located, he immediately has two drinks. Not one. He wants a quick effect and one is not enough. If he is unlucky enough to be invited to a Baptist wedding with the reception in the social hall of the church, precluding alcohol, he doesn't stay long. Or, he has a couple of drinks before the wedding and a flask to keep the buzz going at the reception. I remember vividly in my drinking days I attended a men's retreat at the Mission San Antonio. We were in prayer and discussion groups all day, and at dinner I was surprised that I felt an almost desperate desire for a beer. As we sat down to eat, I noticed a bottle of jug wine on the table. I used to collect good wine, but I had no appetite for bulk wine. In spite of that, I had several glasses to satisfy my craving. I just wanted the alcohol, and it did make me feel better, although I was disgusted with myself for so desperately needing those drinks. It was ten years before I could finally summon the personal and spiritual strength to banish alcohol from my life.

Have you had blackouts after drinking?

There was a young man in my fraternity who literally became psychotic when he was drunk. Chris Putnam was six feet two and 220 pounds without an ounce of fat, and he had been recruited to play center for our top-rated college football team. He was in my pledge class in the fraternity and it was our responsibility to keep him in check when he drank. It was an impossible job. After a number of beers, Chris would become a one-man wrecking crew, throwing chairs through windows, putting his fist through walls, and wrestling with anyone he could get his hands on. It was terrifying to see him on the rampage. I remember several of the bigger and more sober brothers frequently knocking Chris unconscious just to end the siege.

The next morning, Chris was a lamb and he had no recollection of the night before. Having never been so drunk that I couldn't remember my actions, I thought that he was copping out. He wasn't. I've since learned that many young men and women experience blackouts when they drink heavily. The conventional wisdom is that such episodes are not a sign of serious alcoholism and that young people grow out of these phases. This is wrong thinking. If a person has a seizure, we put them on medication to prevent future seizures and we rescind their driver's license to prevent injury to themselves or others. Why should we be more lenient with the alcoholic who has blackouts? Anyone who gets drunk, gets violent, and can't remember the episode should consider their drinking life threatening and seek help immediately.

If you answered yes to one or more of the above, you are an alcoholic. You are not alone. Between 15 and 30 percent of men and 10 to 15 percent of women will answer yes to one of the above, accepted criteria for alcoholism. There are, however, more subtle indications of a growing problem. Answer yes or no to the following:

Can you have just one drink?

Or does one drink make you feel just a tiny bit mellow but you know you'd feel even better if you had another? Or maybe two? The high-functioning alcoholic is in search of that little "buzz," and one drink doesn't get him there. If you drink looking for a "feeling," you are a problem drinker.

Do you drink alone?

If you drink alone, perhaps you are drinking "to relax" after a hard day at work. While there's nothing wrong with that per se, it means you have chosen a chemical form of relaxation that is addictive. You are using alcohol like a drug, a tranquilizer or antianxiety drug. Why not take a Valium or smoke a joint? Anyway you look at it, it's a drug addiction.

You have a problem.

Do you crave a drink?

Does your mouth water at the thought of that first beer? Does your hand tremble as you unscrew the cap, waiting for the ice-cold effervescence? You are conditioned, like Pavlov's dogs. They were reacting to a ringing bell and you're reacting to the concrete representation of a substance that's going to make you feel good. Like a heroin addict who begins to sweat when he heats the mixture in a spoon, your mind and body are anticipating the high. You are kidding yourself if you think it's just a social habit.

It's a drug habit.

Do you drink during the day?

I spent a summer watching a hard-core alcoholic in action. He had his first beer between nine and ten in the morning. He still had a significant blood level of alcohol in his bloodstream from the night before. As it dropped, all the brain chemicals that are dependent on a certain blood concentration of alcohol began to malfunction and Larry became restless and cranky. But after the first couple of beers, he visibly relaxed, and from that point on he drank steadily throughout the day and night.

If you drink during the day, you may be responding to subtle physiological symptoms that are being communicated from your body. Symptoms that are saying, "I'll feel much better if I have a couple of beers." So you do. And you feel better. Unfortunately, you will have to continue to drink during the remainder of your waking hours or you will revert to that edgy feeling.

If this is you, you need to stop.

Do you drive drunk?

Do you drive after drinking more than three or four ounces of alcohol within several hours? The California Highway Patrol estimates that on major urban freeways and road systems after dark, 5 percent, or one in twenty, of all drivers on the road are legally drunk. Legally drunk is a blood alcohol of 0.08 percent. For my height and weight (6 feet 1, 180 pounds), that's three beers. A beer is an ounce of alcohol. Your liver can metabolize alcohol to acetaldehyde at a rate of one ounce per hour. If you drink more than that, your blood level climbs until you stop or pass out.

Driving drunk is a learned skill. It is amazing how the nervous system can adjust to intoxication. Many people who drink a lot can drive reasonably well when they can barely stand, with a blood level of 0.2 percent, for example. And so they do it.

Have you?

You avoid freeways and drive surface streets where there is less scrutiny. You deliberately go the speed limit or slightly slower so as not to attract attention. But driving too slowly or speeding will draw equal attention. Add just the least little weave and you may be blowing into a Breathalyzer. Ironically, good drunk drivers are usually excellent sober drivers and, as a result, rarely get caught. But every now and then they slip up. A good friend was pulled over for a burned-out taillight, not for impaired driving, but the CHP immediately recognized he'd been drinking. He failed a field sobriety test and a Breathalyzer, as his blood alcohol was 0.18 percent. He spent a night in jail and lost his license for six months.

Another friend used to joke that he was a better driver drunk than most other people were sober, remarking that elderly drivers have bad eyesight, have slow reaction times, and are dangerously timid or slow. What he is not acknowledging is that his reaction time in an emergency is three or four times longer drunk than it is sober. The ability to brake in a timely manner, avoid obstacles on the road, and avoid other vehicles is dangerously altered. He is a menace to himself and those in his vehicle, and a threat to everyone around him. But being self-absorbed is a common trait of an alcoholic, so rarely do the safety or rights of other individuals enter into his thinking. He is also ignoring the fact that driving while intoxicated is against the law. Fifty thousand highway fatalities occur each year, equaling the total number of deaths resulting from the Vietnam War (Vietnam War Casualties). When eight of our servicemen die in a training exercise, the entire nation mourns. But 150 deaths on the highway occur every day in this country. In 80 percent of those deaths, alcohol has played a role. And so a wounded nation, seeking to protect itself, set an arbitrary and low limit of 0.08 percent as legally drunk. If you are caught, you will get busted. There is a zero-tolerance rule in the evaluation of highway drunkenness.

And that is as it should be.

Do you say things when you're drinking that you later regret?

Alcohol loosens tongues. We all have many conversations going on in our minds at any given time. There is the reality conversation—taking in the scene around us, evaluating it, and reacting. But simultaneously we have tangential thoughts—some critical, some angry, some frankly paranoid—vying for our attention. We have all had thoughts we were ashamed of, which we know are untrue. When we are sober, we keep these thoughts in check. When we're drunk, often they just come out: "You know, I've been meaning to tell you this for a long time. Your mother is a meddling pain in the ass," or "You've really put on weight," or "Why can't you get good grades like Randy?" And at the time, you may not realize it, but you have pulled the pin out of a hand grenade and it's set to go off. The problem is the next morning you may not even remember having said it. But he or she will. And you can't take it back.

It's not you talking; it's the alcohol.

But it's out there. It's been said. You can only hope that the wounds are not fatal to one you love or to a relationship you cherish. So you bind the wounds and you ask forgiveness and you let healing occur.

You need to be aware that alcohol can amplify any anger in you and it will hurt you and the ones you love. It's not worth the buzz to lose control this way.

Do you do things when you're drinking that you later regret?

Just as alcohol loosens tongues, it also dissolves restraint. Imagine awakening in a strange bed and realizing with horror that you've slept with the unfamiliar body beside you. And since you were drunk enough to have sex with someone you don't know, there's little chance you took any precautions to prevent pregnancy or a sexually transmitted disease. As a result, the incidence of genital herpes simplex is nearly 50 percent in people under thirty. How many unwanted pregnancies, sexually transmitted diseases, and cases of HIV infection are the result of intoxication?

On college campuses, date rape is a familiar occurrence. The male plies his date with alcohol, trying to weaken her resistance. If he has miscalculated her desires or she's not sufficiently inebriated when he initiates sex, she may resist. Fortified with alcohol, he may force her into sex. And if he's really a mean drunk or underestimates his strength, she may be badly hurt or even killed.

Several years ago at our local college, a beautiful young girl disappeared the night after her last final exam. She was seen at a post-finals party rather drunk and was walked back to campus by a young man who said he left her at the end of the walk that led to her dorm. She was never seen again. Corpse-sniffing dogs led police investigators to the young man's dorm room and to his bed, but that evidence is not admissible in court. Her body has never been found and the circumstances of her disappearance have never been explained. Interestingly enough, the young man refused to cooperate with investigators and was never formally charged, but he has shown up several times since in the local police log for drunk driving. For the girl's family and friends, there will be a lifetime of grief, pain, and uncertainty, all due to the devastating effect of alcohol.

The alcohol-induced loss of self-control also applies to the tendency toward physical violence. It is all too common that drunken husbands beat their spouses. National statistics estimate that in 50 percent of all domestic dispute homicides, one or both of the parties are drunk.

Have you ever lost your temper because you were drunk? Have you ever had sex with someone drunk whom you never would have had sex with sober? Have you ever had to apologize for your actions while you were drinking?

You have a problem.

Have you had a sexual failure due to alcohol?

In small amounts, alcohol releases inhibitions and increases animation. That's why it is the drug of choice for people with social anxiety. The ordinarily quiet person becomes loquacious. Alcohol in low doses also increases sexual arousal, but most of us keep on drinking through and past the point of arousal.

This is not nearly as troublesome for the female, as she doesn't need physiological arousal to have sex. For the male, it's much more difficult. He needs to achieve an erection and an orgasm. Both are physiological responses that require good nerve function, and alcohol can dramatically suppress that.

At higher levels of intoxication, say 0.15 to 0.25 percent, many men cannot achieve or maintain an erection. The nerves of the penis, under a complicated and delicate control, cause a dilation of the deep dorsal vein of the shaft, which engorges the tissues, producing a firm and satisfying erection. Many subtle health changes can affect this. Narrowing of arteries due to cigarette smoking, uncontrolled high blood pressure, diabetes, elevated blood cholesterol and/or triglycerides, and the side effects of many prescription medications all compromise the circulation to the penis and jeopardize erections. The shocking revelation that 30 percent or more men at the age of fifty are unable to achieve or maintain erections is evidence of the delicate balance that good circulatory health requires for adequate sexual function. And the male ego is ever so sensitive to the issue of sexual performance. Most men will not admit that they have a problem. The makers of Viagra learned that very quickly. They found that they could vastly increase sales if they let the word slip out that Viagra gives "normal"-functioning men an even firmer, more intense, and longer-lasting erection than if they only marketed it for the FDA-approved use of "erectile dysfunction."

Then, add alcohol to this precarious and highly charged physical and psycho-social scenario. The depressant effect of alcohol on nerves may further wreak havoc on the engorgement process and produce the dreaded failure to erect. After spending thousands of dollars at the urologist's office doing hormone assays and blood-flow studies, does the doctor address the correlation between alcohol con-sumption and reduced sexual function?

A problem equal to erectile dysfunction is failure to achieve orgasm. Orgasm also requires a fully functioning set of pelvic and penile nerves. Adequate sensa-tion of the penile skin is necessary for arousal, and the higher centers of the brain likewise must be in reasonably good health for orgasms to occur. At moderate to high levels of intoxication, there is a general numbing of the sexual skin to the subtle and delicate stimulation required to produce orgasm. At lower blood alco-hol levels, this may prolong orgasm and be beneficial in satisfying the female part-ner. At the higher levels, it may be exhausting to the female partner, since the male can't finish the job.

The higher centers of the brain may also play a role in orgasmic dysfunction. Depression of these centers brought about by higher levels of alcohol may greatly reduce a man's orgasmic ability.

With the many overlapping physical problems that produce sexual dysfunc-tion, it is no wonder that one in three fifty-year-olds are incapable of erection and/or orgasm. Resultant fear of failure adds to the mix. Oftentimes, the woman only observes a decreased frequency of sexual intimacy and what appears to be a loss of interest that is attributed to age.

For the woman, engorgement of the breasts and vulvar tissues is dependent on good nerve function just as it is with the male. Because women can perform sexu-ally without these tissues being fully functional, it is much more difficult to deter-mine the degree of sexual dysfunction attributable to alcohol. The only quantifiable response is orgasm, and since a significant percentage of women are nonorgasmic, or not consistently orgasmic, evaluating the effect of underlying medical illnesses and alcohol on sexual abilities remains a challenge.

In females, as in males, low levels of alcohol may decrease inhibitions and increase arousal. Many women report that they are more readily aroused and achieve orgasm more consistently with a small intake of alcohol. Many will also admit that when they are moderately intoxicated, they are incapable of orgasm.

If you have experienced a change in your sexual capability lately, it may be due to your drinking.

Do you conceal the amount you drink from your friends or significant other?

One excellent strategy to force a person to recognize that he has a significant problem with alcohol is to count the number of ounces of alcohol he consumes. Confronted with the actual volume of intoxicant, many heavy drinkers are unable to deny that they have a problem.

The drinker in denial, however, goes to great lengths to conceal the actual amount he is drinking. If he drinks hard liquor, he may have a secret stash from which he refills the bottle in the cupboard so that it is not apparent how much he really consumes. The wine drinker may have two or three bottles in the fridge and tipples from all of them so that the amount consumed is not readily apparent. Beer drinkers have a spare six-pack or two in the cupboard and replace each one as it is drunk so that the fridge always looks full. Having several different brands on hand also helps to confuse the issue.

If you conduct this kind of alcoholic sleight of hand, you have a problem.

Do you refuse to answer the phone in the evening because your speech is slightly slurred?

After three to four ounces of alcohol, there are some very subtle changes in speech patterns. Words are transposed, memory is ever so slightly impaired, and there is a slurring of certain words. Having been a high-functioning alcoholic, and recalling a lifetime of phone conversations with my parents who drank heavily every night, I have a sensitively trained ear for intoxicated speech. I could also detect it in my own speech at a very early stage. As I aged, I was amazed at changes in my speech after ingesting little alcohol. Just two or three beers would produce slight speech alterations and memory lapses (rationalized as "senior moments") that were very frightening. I began to worry that I was developing early Alzheimer's dementia. I had also sustained several severe head injuries, and it wasn't entirely clear whether or not some of the changes were part of a post-concussion syndrome. Since I was at a stage where I neither wanted to nor could stop drinking, I just wouldn't answer the phone in the evening, for fear that the person on the other end of the line could detect my intoxication.

In retrospect, some of the memory and cognitive impairment may have been simple fatigue. My workdays are long and intense, leaving me physically and mentally drained at times.

Miraculously, five years after quitting, my memory is almost perfect, and my concerns about the late sequelae of head trauma are lessened. But I am acutely aware of other people's speech patterns and hypersensitive to the subtle signs of intoxication in speech and thinking. And I am astounded at the number of people I talk to on the phone at night who sound drunk.

Does this sound familiar?

Do you use mints or mouthwash to cover the smell of alcohol on your breath?

Doubtless because I have had my own issues with alcohol, I am extremely aware of what I sense to be problems in others. High-functioning alcoholics are usually pretty cagey, though, and some are paranoid or ashamed enough to want to hide the problem from others. Like some smokers who take a SenSen to hide the smoke on their breath, many drinkers are acutely aware that alcohol is readily detectable on the breath. They have breath mints in pocket or purse or carry one of those little spray bottles of mouthwash in the car or on their person.

This is premeditation. It means that they drink regularly and seek to cover it up, a sign of a serious problem.

Is this you?

Are you disgusted with yourself every morning because you drank last night?

Problem drinkers, unless totally brain-dead, know deep inside that they are addicted. And it disgusts them. No one likes to feel out of control, enslaved by anyone or anything. So they wake up in the morning and feel awful, not from being hungover (most chronic drinkers have adjusted to that) but from being unhappy with themselves. They may have insight; they may not. The fact that they do feel terrible is a sure sign they have a problem. But it's also a ray of hope. Disgust can be a powerful motive for quitting once the realization comes and the will is mobilized.

Are you tired of being a slave to alcohol?

Reread the preceding questions and answer yes or no to each one. Be honest with yourself. If you have one question answered affirmatively, you have a drinking problem and you are heading for a bigger one in the future. It is time to admit it and look for help.

34

FREE AT LAST: HOW I GOT SOBER AND HOW IT CHANGED MY LIFE

Okay, so it didn't just happen. I didn't just wake up on Ash Wednesday, 2001, and miraculously stop drinking. I did stop drinking, but there needed to be intellectual, spiritual, and physical strategies in place to bolster my resolve. They were the product of countless failed attempts and a complete resignation of my personal strength and will to God.

Simple, but not easy.

Intellectually, I could see the person I had become. What was it that the kid had said? "Some drunk grabbed me by the neck." It was my first real public performance as a mean drunk. My worst fears had come true. I was acting just like my dad when he drank. There was such shame and public humiliation. Continuing to behave like that was intolerable to my sense of who I really was. That wasn't me. I am not that mean drunk. (Oh yes I was.)

In recovery they say that some people have to hit bottom before they "get it," before they have the moment of clarity that allows them to see, finally, what a mess alcohol has made of their lives. The guys in my Friday night group think that I had the highest bottom of any alcoholic they know. That's all right with me. I didn't have to retch up half my blood volume or kill someone on the freeway. That is perfectly okay with me. Intellectually, I got the message.

Spiritually, I had been preparing myself for a long time. My search for the presence of God and how He fit in my life had produced some dramatic, life-altering insights. I discovered that there was a hole in my soul that left me very empty and that robbed my life of the meaning that I knew I needed to find peace and happiness. I found that God was the only thing that could fill that void. In my Christian teaching, it was the Holy Spirit, God's presence in me, His gift to His children when He reclaimed His son from earth; that was the only thing that would fit. Since I was baptized, I had been given the gift of the Holy Spirit, but instead of being a conflagration that fired me from within, it was a tiny little Bunsen burner whose light was barely visible. I wanted more. I wanted a rocket engine. As my spiritual desire grew, so did my frustration. Until my epiphany: alcohol and true spirituality do not mix. There is no room for the Holy Spirit in the soul that is continually under the influence.

I had to choose. I decided on the path that would lead me home to God. Sober.

Physically, I knew the intellectual and the spiritual would not succeed unless I could keep myself from lifting an ice-cold beer to my lips. That was the challenge. I had some insights from years of drinking and failed attempts to quit. I knew that I craved the high I got with alcohol, but I also realized that part of the relief I felt when I drank was the rapid correction of a low blood sugar. Remember, ethanol functions as a two-carbon sugar. It is absorbed right through the mucosae of the mouth, esophagus, stomach, and intestine. It doesn't need to be transported into the intestine or digested. It's instantaneous. So part of the physical benefit of drinking, say at the end of a long workday, was getting my blood sugar up where I felt good. The first physical change I had to make was to find something else to take its place. I tried carrots and they worked. When I come home at night, I feed the horses. They always get a couple of carrots in their feed buckets. I buy a twenty-five-pound bag of juicing carrots twice a week at the store. They are the size of Little League bats, but they are surprisingly sweet and work as well as two Budweisers. When I ran out of carrots, I tried drinking a glass of milk, eating some cheese, and eating an energy bar, all of which worked very well.

Over the past five years, I have learned to carry an energy bar in my briefcase, and I have cheese in the fridge at the office. I never let my blood sugar get too low. It has greatly diminished the craving for alcohol. I also have learned that if I am sober, I am much less likely to experience hypoglycemia. Alcohol prevents the liver from storing glycogen (long chains of glucose), which can be released to buffer an episode of hypoglycemia.

My knowledge of diminishing cravings really helped my abstinence. So, I knew if I could make it a week or two without drinking, I would have a good chance of finally quitting.

So, armed with the repugnant, intolerable mental image of myself as a mean, abusive drunk, and with pockets stuffed with energy bars and carrots, I entered

Lent, 2001, by asking God to take over, to do what I could not. After a week, it became physically easier, and the sacred fire of the Holy Spirit has become such a precious gift for me that I would never give it up for the physical pleasure of drinking a beer.

Once sober, I began to see that was not enough. I needed to know what it was that made me need to drink, to get drunk, and to be addicted. One of my mentors, Bud Beecher, loaned me *Adult Children of Alcoholics*, by Timmen Cermak, MD. There, I read a psychological portrait of myself. So many things made sense. It is beyond the scope of this book to go into the many dynamics of the ACA, but I am gradually coming to grips with the way I was raised and the profound effect it continues to have on me.

I did not gain sobriety as a member of a group, but I have been to meetings and I enjoy the company of the brave and honest men and women that I find there. I would never have envisioned myself in organized recovery, but I appreciate the fellowship of so many remarkable men with decades of sobriety. Some of these wise old owls have profound insights into alcoholism and a venerable sense of calm contentedness that is a cherished goal for my life. Almost every week there is someone with less than thirty days of sobriety, someone who has "been out" and is trying to get back in. Seeing those struggling souls, I silently thank God for His gift of my sobriety.

Most organized recovery programs are built on a twelve-step program that has the potential to transform one's life. AA's can be found in the appendix of this book. The twelve steps are the blueprint for a spiritual awakening from which anyone, sober or not, could benefit. I progressed through the first three steps on my own; the difficult ones await. Admitting all my wrongs to another person, revealing the dark episodes of my drunken past, and then making amends, where possible, is a challenge that will test my belief in a loving God and in his forgiveness. I am sure the steps were created to produce exactly that circumstance. It will be as hard as getting sober. But, contentment and inner peace will be the reward.

In sobriety, it is said you have to change everything about your life. That's not always true. When you get sober, everything will change around you as it did for me. I've been married for twenty years and my wife likes me much better sober. She never drank much and drinks even less now, and she is very supportive of my mission to wake up as many people as possible to the disaster alcohol can create for them. The most significant change is that many of my old friends have drifted away. Most of them drink, some a lot, and my sobriety is threatening to them, so they prefer not to have me at their parties. That's okay with me. I miss them and their friendships, but at least two have gotten sober since I did, and now we have even more in common.

I lost my dad last fall to gastric carcinoma, a cancer known to be caused by alcohol and tobacco, both of which he abused. He was a dear, sweet man whom I loved unreservedly, but his high-functioning alcoholism of five decades deteriorated in the last fifteen years of his life. White wine and vodka salved the aches and pains and the grief of aging. He knew I was sober but he didn't really know how I felt about his drinking. It was just one more in a multitude of denials.

My mother lives in a quiet senior residence. She drinks a lot less than she did when Dad was alive. Like him, she is not consciously aware that their lives were dominated by drinking, or how it affected me and my siblings.

Both my sisters drink but not to excess. They are aware of our parents' problem but don't, as yet, understand the profound ways such an upbringing has affected them. They both understand and support my recovery, for which I am grateful.

The most profound change is my delight at learning who I am sober and discovering that I genuinely love the person I am becoming. Thomas Merton speaks of the true self. I am becoming my true self. There is a sense of awe and gratitude in that. I praise God that I can experience peace and happiness I didn't think possible and that the hole in my soul is filled with a fire that, I pray, will light the darkness for brothers and sisters who suffer as I did.

> *"And be not drunk with wine, wherein is excess;*
> *but be filled with the Holy Spirit."*
> *Ephesians 5:18 (KJV)*

35

WHY SHOULD YOU QUIT?

○ ○

"You speak to me of sadness
and the coming of the winter.
The fear that is within you now
that seems to never end.
The dreams that have escaped you
And the hope that you'd forgotten.
You tell me that you need me now
You want to be my friend.
You wonder where we're going
Where's the rhyme and where's the reason."

—*John Denver*

He couldn't find the lever that engaged the auxiliary gas tank. The plane sputtered, stalled, and dropped into the Pacific like a stone. A generation lost an icon in John Denver.

He always appeared happy and his lyrics spoke of beauty and love, but Denver had a dark side. The "Rocky Mountain High" possessed him for a time. How ironic that he should die so tragically after succeeding against addiction.

I am drawn to the lyric of this song because it speaks to a fear we all share. If we are not persistent, focused, and lucky, many of our dreams will escape us even when sober. If not sober, alcohol and other addictions will surely rob us of those dreams and of the hope that makes life worth living.

Alcoholism is hopeless. Along with the terms "despair" and "slavery," "hopelessness" is another apt description of the wretchedness of addiction to alcohol.

Many who know me do not believe that I am an alcoholic. They believe I never really had a problem with drinking, but they are wrong. They believe this partly because they currently drink as heavily as I did, and if they acknowledge that I have a problem, they would have to admit they have one as well. Additionally, they don't have the insight and awareness of what alcohol was doing to me and what it might be doing to them.

Alcohol made me a different person, someone I don't like as well as the person that I am sober. It made me angry, impatient, and critical. It prevented me from experiencing and expressing the spiritual side of my nature when I was under its influence, which was nearly every day. So in that sense, it certainly was a problem.

I am not the kind of person who can drink one beer twice a week. Sure, I could apply my iron discipline for a week or two or perhaps a month. But one night I'd want two or even three and gradually, after several months, I'd be back to two to four beers six nights a week. And realistically, though I like the little "feel good" that I experience midway through the second beer, I hate the depression that three and four beers create. But, I can't stop with two. I keep trying to recapture the "feel-good" moment.

I wasn't a hard-core alcoholic headed for cirrhosis and varices. But I could have developed neuropathy, sexual dysfunction, and memory problems at the level I was drinking. Since I quit, my memory and my libido have never been better. That's not why I quit, but it surely has been a side benefit.

The bottom line is being completely honest with yourself. If someone followed you all day for a week and wrote a diary of your activities, including your drinking, would you be perfectly comfortable having it published in the local newspaper? What about the drinks you sneak when no one is looking? What about the trip to the liquor store for a six-pack on the way home from work? Those seemingly innocent little dishonesties are the first indication of the immorality that alcohol will eventually produce. It is the beginning of the cancer.

If you ignore it, it can grow and spread.

And it may kill you. Or it may simply rob you of your dreams and of hope.

So often, it takes decades to know the truth. But at least some of us do, eventually. Today I could easily still be drinking and deluding myself. Reading the account of my struggle may or may not bring you to an awakening. But if this window into alcoholism both on a personal level and on a medical level encourages just one person to overcome this disease, it will have accomplished its purpose.

WORKS CITED

Alcoholics Anonymous. (2001). 4th ed. New York: Alcoholics Anonymous World Services.

CDC Fact Book 2001–2. Retrieved from http://www.cdc.gov/ncipc/ fact_book_different.htm

Enzinger, C. et al. "Risk factors for Progression of Brain Atrophy in Aging: Six-Year Follow-Up of Normal Subjects." *Neurology* 64 (May 2005): 1704–1706.

Jefferis, B. J. et al. "Adolescent Drinking Level and Adult Binge Drinking in a National Birth Cohort." *Addiction* 100 (April 2005): 543-549.

Miller, J. W. et al. "Prevalence of Adult Binge Drinking: A Comparison of Two National Surveys." *American Journal of Preventive Medicine* 27(3): 197-204.

Morbidity and Mortality Weekly Report (MMWR). 53(22): 471-474.

Morbidity and Morality Weekly Report (MMWR) 54(2005, April 22): 377-380.

Nadeau, Remi. Fort Laramie and the Sioux. Crest Publishers, Santa Barbara, CA, 1997

Rumbaugh, C. L. et al. *Investigative Radiology* 11(July-August 1976): 282-294.

Anon. University of Pittsburgh School of Medicine, Student Affairs Handbook, 2005 Retrieved from http://www.medschool.pitt.edu/studentaffairs/alcohol.html

Anon. Vietnam War Casualties. 2003 Retrieved from http://www.vietnamwar-info/casualties/

APPENDIX A

Alcohol and Immunity

Enzinger, C. et al. "Risk factors for Progression of Brain Atrophy in Aging: Six-Year Follow-Up of Normal Subjects." *Neurology* 64 (May 2005):1704–1706.

Gonzalez-Quintana, A. "Alcohol Increases IGE Levels." *Alcohol Clin Exp Rev* 26 (2002): 60–64.

Wang, Y. "Vit E Blocks Alcohol-Induced Immune Suppression." *Alcohol Clin Exp Rev* 18(2): 355–362.

Grossman, C. J. "Alcohol Decreases Maturation of Thymic T Cells." *Int J Immunopharmacol* 10(2): 187–195.

Chang, M. P. "Alcohol Suppresses T Lymphocyte Proliferation." *Int J Immunopharmacol* 14(4): 707–719

Na, H. R. "Alcohol Suppresses Cell-Mediated Immunity." *Alcohol Clin Exp Rev* 21(7): 1179–1185.

Wu, W. J. "Alcohol Decreases Natural Killer T Cells." *Int J Cancer* 82(6): 886–892.

Alcohol and Cancer

Wu, W. J. "Alcohol Decreases Host Resistance to Spread of Melanoma." *Int J Cancer* 82(6): 886–892.

Mufti, S. J. "Alcohol Promotes Cancer of the Gastrointestinal Tract." *Cancer Detect Prev* 22(3): 195–203.

Thun, M. J. "Alcohol Increases Death Rate from Breast Cancer by 30 Percent." *N Engl J Med* 337(24): 1705–1714.

Thomas, D. B. "Alcohol and Tobacco Account for 80 Percent of Cancer of the Mouth, Pharynx, Larynx, and Esophagus in the United States." *Environ Health Perspect* 103(Suppl 8): 153–160.

Schottenfeld, D. "Alcohol Is an Important Factor in Causing Liver Cancer." *Cancer* 43(5 suppl): 1962–1966.

Key, T. J. "Alcohol Increases Risk of Breast Cancer." *Lancet Oncol* 2(3): 133–140.

Wrensch, M. "Alcohol May Be Partially Responsible for Higher Rates of Breast Cancer in Marin County, California, Than Elsewhere." *Breast Cancer Res* 5(4): R88–R102.

Homann, N. "Alcohol's Breakdown Product Acetaldehyde Is Toxic, Mutagenic, and Carcinogenic." *Addict Biol* 6(4): 309–323.

Li, D. "Alcohol May Promote Pancreatic Cancer by Increasing K-ras Mutation." *Cancer J* 7(4): 259–265.

Noda, T. "Alcoholics Have Higher Mortality Rates from *All Cancers*." *Psychiatry Clin Neurosci* 55(5): 466–472.

Novak, R. F. "Alcohol Increases CYP2E1 Variant of Cytochrome P450, Which May Promote Cancer Development." *Arch Pharm Res* 23(4): 267–282.

Fetal Alcohol Syndrome

"Northwest Portland Area Maternal Child Health Newsletter." *Pediatrics* 106(2): 358–360.

Alcohol and Osteoporosis

Nishiguchi, S. "Alcohol Decreases Bone Mineral Density, Greater in Females Than in Males." *J Bone Miner Metab* 18(6): 317–320.

Faine, M. P. "Alcohol Increases Urinary Loss of Calcium." *J Prosthet Dent* 73(1): 65–72.

Ringe, J. D. "Alcohol Is Second Most Important Risk Factor in Osteoporosis in Men." *Dtsch Med Wochenschr* 119(27): 943–947.

Zima, T. "Alcohol Causes Decreased Parathyroid Hormone, Thus Lowering Calcium." *Sb Lek* 94(4): 303–309.

Laitinen, K. "Increased Urinary Excretion of Calcium and Decreased Serum Calcium Are Noted Eight Hours After Alcohol Intake." *N Engl J Med* 324(11): 721–727.

Alcohol and Gastroesophageal Reflux Disease (GERD)

Bujanda, L. "Alcohol Decreases Force of Contraction of Esophageal Muscle and Weakens Sphincter While Increasing Stomach Acid Production." *Am J Gastroenterol* 95(12): 3374–3382.

Kaufman, S. E. "Alcohol Causes GERD." *Gut* 19(4): 336–338.

Vitale, J. C. "Alcohol Significantly Increases the Acidity of the Distal Esophagus by Permitting Increased Reflux of Stomach Acid." *JAMA* 258(15): 2077–2079.

Choy, D. "Gastroesophageal Reflux May Cause Asthma by Stimulating the Vagus Nerve, and Asthma May Cause GERD by Changing Esophageal Dynamics Via Altered Diaphragmatic Movement." *Respirology* 2(3): 163–168.

APPENDIX B

THE TWELVE STEPS OF ALCOHOLICS ANONYMOUS

1. We admitted we were powerless over alcohol—that our lives had become unmanageable.

2. Came to believe that a power greater than ourselves could restore us to sanity.

3. Made a decision to turn our will and our lives over to the care of God *as we understood Him.*

4. Made a searching and fearless moral inventory of ourselves.

5. Admitted to God, to ourselves, and to another human being the exact nature of our wrongs.

6. Were entirely ready to have God remove all these defects of character.

7. Humbly asked Him to remove our shortcomings.

8. Made a list of all persons we had harmed, and became willing to make amends to them all.

9. Made direct amends to such people wherever possible, except when to do so would injure them or others.

10. Continued to take personal inventory and when we were wrong promptly admitted it.

11. Sought through prayer and meditation to improve our conscious contact with God, *as we understood Him*, praying only for knowledge of His will for us and the power to carry that out.

12. Having had a spiritual awakening as a result of these steps, we tried to carry this message to alcoholics and to practice these principles in all our affairs.

978-0-595-37994-
0-595-37994-X

Printed in the United States
78991LV00003B/122